Kṛṣṇa Consciousness

The Topmost Yoga System

Books by His Divine Grace
A.C. Bhaktivedanta Swami Prabhupāda:

Bhagavad-gītā As It Is
Śrīmad-Bhāgavatam
(18 vols.; with disciples)
Śrī Caitanya-caritāmṛta (9 vols.)
Kṛṣṇa, The Supreme Personality
of Godhead
Teachings of Lord Caitanya
The Nectar of Devotion
The Nectar of Instruction
Śrī Īśopaniṣad
Light of the Bhāgavata
Easy Journey to Other Planets
The Science of Self-Realization
Kṛṣṇa Consciousness: The Topmost
Yoga System
Perfect Questions, Perfect Answers
Teachings of Lord Kapila, the Son of
Devahuti
Transcendental Teachings of Prahlāda
Mahārāja
Teachings of Queen Kuntī
Kṛṣṇa, the Reservoir of Pleasure
The Path of Perfection
Life Comes from Life
Message of Godhead
The Perfection of Yoga
Beyond Birth and Death
On the Way to Kṛṣṇa
Rāja-vidyā: The King of Knowledge
Elevation to Kṛṣṇa Consciousness
Kṛṣṇa Consciousness:
The Matchless Gift
The Nārada-bhakti-sūtra (with disciples)
The Mukunda-mālā-stotra
(with disciples)
A Second Chance
The Journey of Self-Discovery
The Laws of Nature
Renunciation through Wisdom
Civilization & Transcendence
The Quest for Enlightenment
Beyond Illusion and Doubt
Dharma: The way of Transcendence
Introduction to Bhagavad-gītā
The Hare Krishna Challenge
Geetār-gan (Bengali)
Vairāgya-vidyā (Bengali)
Buddhi-yoga (Bengali)
Bhakti-ratna-bolī (Bengali)
Back to Godhead magazine (founder)

A complete catalogue is available upon request.
The Bhaktivedanta Book Trust, Hare Krishna Land, Juhu, Mumbai 400 049.
The above books are available at ISKCON centres too. Please contact a centre near you for your requirements.

Kṛṣṇa Consciousness

The Topmost Yoga System

His Divine Grace
A.C. Bhaktivedanta Swami Prabhupāda
Founder-Ācārya of the International Society for Krishna Consciousness

THE BHAKTIVEDANTA BOOK TRUST

Readers interested in the subject matter of this book are invited by The Bhaktivedanta Book Trust to correspond with its Secretary at the following address:

The Bhaktivedanta Book Trust
Hare Krishna Land,
Juhu, Mumbai 400 049, India.

E-mail: bbtmumbai@pamho.net
Web: www.bbtindia.net

Previous printings in India: 70,000 copies
Tenth printing, September 2004: 20,000 copies

Published by Bhima dasa for The Bhaktivedanta Book Trust-Mumbai and printed at Magna Graphics (India) Ltd., Kandivali (West), Mumbai- 400 067.

Contents

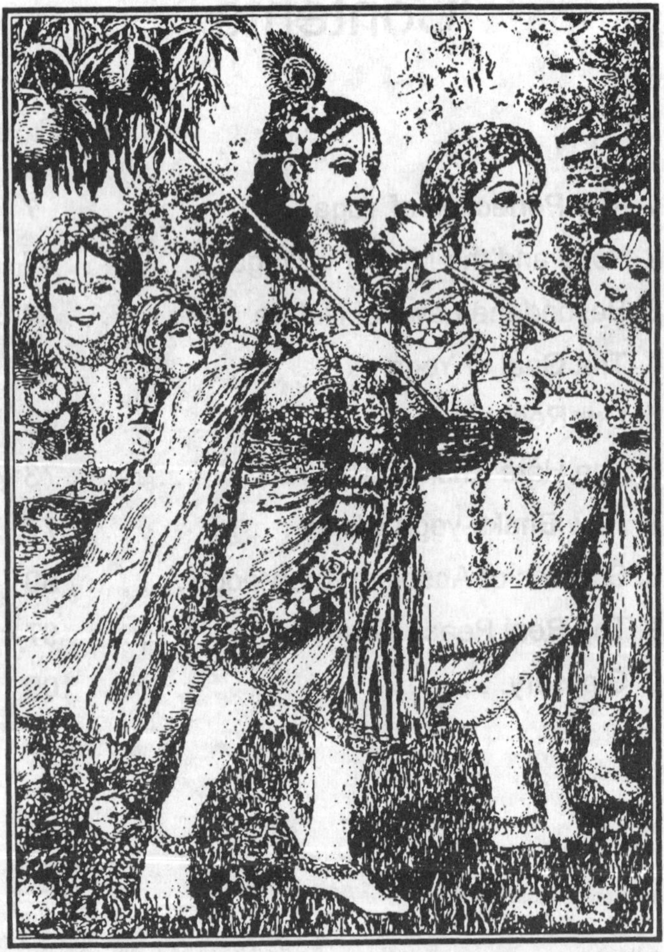

1

The Perfection of Yoga

Lord Kṛṣṇa, the Supreme Personality of Godhead, speaks about the topmost system of *yoga* in the Sixth Chapter of *Bhagavad-gītā.* There He has explained the *haṭha-yoga* system. Please remember that we are preaching this Kṛṣṇa consciousness movement on the authority of *Bhagavad-gītā.* It is nothing manufactured. The *bhakti-yoga* system is authorized, and if you want to know about God, then you have to adopt this *bhakti-yoga* system because in the Sixth Chapter of *Bhagavad-gītā* it is concluded that the topmost *yogī* is he who is always thinking of Kṛṣṇa within himself.

Kṛṣṇa, the supreme authority, recommended the eightfold *yoga* system. The first step of this *yoga* system is to select a very secluded and sacred place. Eightfold meditation cannot be performed in a fashionable city. It is not possible. In India, therefore, those who are very serious about practicing *yoga* go to Hardwar, a very secluded place in the Himalayas, where they remain alone and follow a very restrictive process for eating and sleeping. There is no question of mating. Those rules and regulations must be followed very strictly. Simply to make a show of gymnastics is not perfection of *yoga. Yoga* means control of the senses. If you indulge your senses unrestrictedly but make a show of *yoga* practice, you will never be successful. You have to select a sacred place; then you have to sit with half-closed eyes and concentrate on the tip of your nose. You cannot change your posture. There are many rules and regulations which cannot possibly be followed at the present.

Even 5,000 years ago, when circumstances in the world were different, this *yoga* system was not practicable. Even such a great personality as Arjuna, who belonged to the royal family and was a great warrior and an intimate friend of Kṛṣṇa's, constantly living with Him, after hearing this process of *yoga* from Kṛṣṇa in a face-to-face discussion, said, "My dear Kṛṣṇa, it is not possible to follow." He flatly admitted, "For me these rules and regulations and practice for controlling the mind are not possible." We have to think, then: 5,000 years ago a personality like Arjuna expressed his inability to practice this eightfold *yoga* system, so how can we follow it now?

In this age people are very short-lived. In India the average duration of life is thirty-five years. In your country it may be more than that. But actually, whereas your grandfather lived for 100 years, you cannot. These things are changing. The duration of life will be reduced. There are predictions in the scriptures that in this age, man's duration of life, his mercy and his intelligence are being reduced. Men are not very powerful; their duration of life is very short. We are always disturbed, and we have practically no knowledge about spiritual science.

For example, in the hundreds and thousands of universities all over the world there is no department of knowledge where the science of the soul is taught. Actually, we are all spirit soul. From *Bhagavad-gītā* we understand that we are transmigrating from one body to another, even in our present lives. All of us had at one time the body of a small baby. Where is that body? That body is gone. Presently I am an old man, but I remember that I was once a small baby. I still remember when I was about six months old; I was lying down on the lap of my elder sister, who was knitting, and I was playing. I can remember that, so it is possible for everyone to remember that he had a small body. After the baby's body I had a boy's body; then I had a youthful body, and now I am in this body. Where are those bodies? They are gone now. This is a different body. It is explained in *Bhagavad-gītā* that when I give up this body, I will have to accept another body. It is very simple to understand. I have changed so many bodies, not only from childhood to boyhood to youth, but according to medical science we are changing bodies every second, imperceptibly. This process indicates that the soul is permanent. Although I have changed many bodies, I remember my baby body and my childhood body–I am the same person, soul. Similarly, when ultimately I change this body, I shall have to accept another. This simple formula is stated in *Bhagavad-gītā.* Everyone can reflect on it, and there must be scientific research done in this area.

Recently I received a letter from a doctor in Toronto. He suggested that there is body and there is soul. I corresponded with him. Actually, it is a fact. The soul is there. There is so much evidence, not only in the Vedic literature but even by ordinary experience. The soul is there, and it is transmigrating from one body to another, but unfortunately there is no serious study on this subject in the universities. This is not very good. The *Vedānta-sūtra* says, "This human form of life is meant for searching out the spirit, the Absolute Truth." The *yoga* system is used to search out the spiritual principles within this material world. That process for searching is recommended in *Bhagavad-gītā* by Kṛṣṇa Himself. When Arjuna said, "The system You are recommending, the *haṭha-yoga* system, is not possible for me," Kṛṣṇa assured him that he was the greatest of all *yogīs*. He pacified him by saying not to bother about being unable to practice *haṭha-yoga*. He told him, "Of all different types of *yogīs—haṭha-yogīs, jñāna-yogīs, dhyāna-yogīs, bhakta-yogīs, karma-yogīs*—you are the best *yogī*." Kṛṣṇa says, "Of all *yogīs,* the one who is constantly thinking of Me within himself, meditating upon Me within the heart, is the first-class *yogī.*"

Who can think of Kṛṣṇa always within himself? This is very easy to understand. If you love someone, you can think of him always within you; otherwise it is not possible. If you love someone, then naturally you think of him always. That is described in the *Brahma-saṁhitā.* One who has developed love of God, Kṛṣṇa, can think of Him constantly. When I speak of Kṛṣṇa you should understand that He is God. Another name for Kṛṣṇa is Śyāmasundara, which means that He is blackish like a cloud but very beautiful. In one verse of *Brahma-saṁhitā* it is said that a *santa,* a saintly person, who has developed love for Syāmasundara, Kṛṣṇa, thinks of the Lord constantly within his heart. Actually, when one comes to the point of *samādhi* in the *yoga* system, he thinks, without cessation, of the Viṣṇu form of the Lord within the heart. He is absorbed in that thought.

Kṛṣṇa, Śyāmasundara, is the original Viṣṇu. That is stated in *Bhagavad-gītā.* Kṛṣṇa includes Brahmā, Viṣṇu, Śiva and everyone else. According to Vedic scripture, He expands first as Baladeva, Baladeva expands as Saṅkarṣaṇa, Saṅkarṣaṇa expands as Nārāyaṇa, and Nārāyaṇa expands as Viṣṇu (Mahā-Viṣṇu, Garbodakśāyī Viṣṇu and Kṣīrodakaśāyī Viṣṇu). These are Vedic statements. We can understand that Kṛṣṇa is the original Viṣṇu, Śyāmasundara.

This is the perfect system. Anyone who is thinking of Kṛṣṇa always within himself is a first-class *yogī.* If you want perfection in *yoga,* don't be satisfied only by practicing codes. You have to go further. Actually, the perfection of *yoga* is reached when you are in *samādhi,* always thinking of the Viṣṇu form of the Lord within your heart, without being disturbed. Therefore *yogīs* go to a secluded place, and by controlling all the senses and the mind and concentrating everything on the form of Viṣṇu, they reach *samādhi.* That is called perfection of *yoga.* Actually this *yoga* system is very, very difficult. It may be possible for some solitary man, but for the general mass of people it is not recommended in the scriptures: *harer nāma harer nāma harer nāmaiva kevalam/ kalau nāsty eva nāsty eva nāsty eva gatir anyathā.* "In this age of Kali one must chant the holy names of the

Lord for deliverance. There is no other alternative. There is no other alternative. There is no other alternative." *(Bṛhan-Nāradīya Purāṇa)*

The *yoga* system, as it was recommended in the Satya-yuga, the Golden Age, was to always meditate on Viṣṇu. In the Treta-yuga one could practice *yoga* by performing great sacrifices, and in the next age, Dvāpara-yuga, one could achieve perfection by temple worship. The present age is called Kali-yuga. Kali-yuga means the age of quarrel and disagreement. No one agrees with anyone else. Everyone has his own theory; everyone has his own philosophy. If I don't agree with you, you fight me. This is the symptom of Kali-yuga. The only method recommended in this age is chanting the holy name. Simply by chanting the holy name of God, one can attain that perfect self-realization which was attained by the *yoga* system in the Satya-yuga, by performance of great sacrifices in the Treta-yuga, and by large-scale temple worship in the Dvāpara-yuga. That perfection can be attained by the simple method of *Hari kīrtana. Hari* means the Supreme Personality of Godhead; *kīrtana* means to glorify.

This method is recommended in the scriptures, and it was given to us by Caitanya Mahāprabhu 500 years ago. He appeared in a town which is known as Navadvīpa. It is about sixty miles north of Calcutta. People still go there. We have a temple center there. It is also a sacred place of pilgrimage. Caitanya Mahāprabhu appeared there, and He started this mass *saṅkīrtana* movement, which is conducted without discrimination. He predicted that this *saṅkīrtana* movement would be spread all over the world and that the Hare Kṛṣṇa *mantra* would be chanted in every village and town on the surface of the globe. In pursuance of the order of Lord Caitanya Mahāprabhu, following in His footsteps, we are trying to introduce this *saṅkīrtana* movement, chanting Hare Kṛṣṇa, and it is proving very successful everywhere. I am preaching especially in foreign countries, all over Europe, America, Japan, Canada, Australia, Malaysia, etc. I have introduced this *saṅkīrtana* movement, and now we have centers around the world. All eighty centers are being received with great enthusiasm. I have not imported these boys and girls from India, but they are taking this movement very seriously because it appeals to the soul directly.

We have different stages of our life–the bodily concept of life, the mental concept of life, the intellectual concept of life, and the spiritual concept of life. Actually we are concerned with the spiritual concept. Those who are allured by the bodily concept are no better than cats and dogs. If we accept that "I am this body," then we are not better than the cats and dogs because their concept of life is like that. We must understand that "I am not this body," as Kṛṣṇa wanted to impress upon Arjuna in the beginning of His teaching of *Bhagavad-gītā:* "First of all, try to understand what you are. Why are you lamenting in the bodily concept of life? You have to fight. Certainly you have to fight with your brothers, brothers-in-law and nephews, and you are lamenting. But first of all understand whether you are body or not." That is the beginning of *Bhagavad-gītā*. Kṛṣṇa tried to make Arjuna understand that he was not his body. This instruction was not for Arjuna exclusively, but for everyone. First of all we have to learn that "I am not this body," that "I am spirit soul." That is Vedic instruction.

As soon as you come to this point of being firmly convinced that you are not this body, that is called the *brahma-bhūta* stage of Brahman realization. That is knowledge, real knowledge. Advancement of knowledge for eating, sleeping and mating is animal knowledge. A dog also knows how to eat, how to sleep, how to mate and how to defend. If our education extends only to these points (the dog is eating according to his nature, and we are also eating, but in a nice place, with nicely cooked food on a nice table). that is not advancement. The principle is still eating. Similarly, you may sleep in a very nice apartment in a six-story building or in a 122-story building, and the dog may lie in a street, but when he sleeps and when you sleep, there is no difference. You cannot know whether you are sleeping in a skyscraper or on the ground because you are dreaming something which has taken you from your bed. You have forgotten that your body is lying there on the bed, and you are flying in the air, dreaming. Therefore, to improve the sleeping method is not advancement of civilization. Similarly, the dog has no social custom for mating. Whenever there is a she-dog, he mates on the street. You may mate very silently, in a secret place (although now people are learning how to mate like dogs), but the mating is there. The same principle applies to defending. A dog has teeth and nails with which he can defend himself, and you have atom bombs. But the purpose is defending, that's all. Therefore, scripture says that human life is not meant only for these four principles of life, bodily demands. There is another thing–a human being should be inquisitive to learn what is Absolute Truth. That education is lacking.

According to Vedic civilization a *brāhmaṇa* is a learned man, or one who knows the spirit. In India, *brāhmanas* are addressed as learned men, but in fact they cannot be *brāhmaṇas* by birth. They are expected to know what is spirit.

By birth everyone is a *śūdra,* a fourth-class man, but he may be reformed by the purificatory process. There are ten kinds of purificatory processes. One undergoes all these processes and at last comes to the spiritual master who gives him the sacred thread as recognition of his second birth. One birth is by your father and mother, and the other birth is by the spiritual master and Vedic knowledge. That is called second birth. At that time the candidate is given a chance to study and understand what is *Veda.* By studying all the *Vedas* very nicely, he actually realizes what is spirit and what is his relationship with God, and then he becomes a *brāhmaṇa.* Above that situation of impersonal Brahman understanding, he comes to the platform of understanding Lord Viṣṇu, the Supreme Personality of Godhead; then he becomes a Vaiṣṇava. This is the perfectional process.

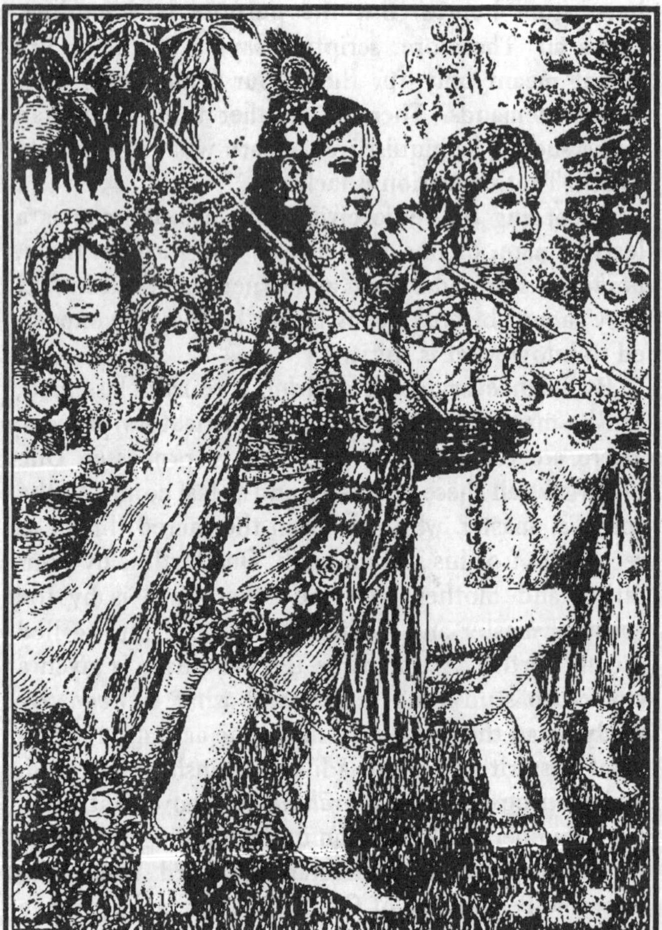

2
Yoga and the Master of Yoga

Yoga means the connecting link between the soul and the Supersoul, or the Supreme and the minute living creatures. Lord Śrī Kṛṣṇa is that Supreme, the Personality of Godhead. Being, therefore, the ultimate object of *yoga,* Kṛṣṇa's name is *yogeśvara,* the master of *yoga.*

At the conclusion of the *Bhagavad-gītā*, it is said: "Where there is Kṛṣṇa, and where there is Arjuna, the greatest of bowmen, there, undoubtedly, is victory."

The *Bhagavad-gītā* is a narrative spoken by Sañjaya, the secretary of Mahārāja Dhṛtarāṣṭra. This is just like airwaves from the radio: the play is going on in the auditorium, but you can hear from your room. So, just as we now have such a mechanical arrangement, at that time there were also certain arrangements, although there was no machine. Anyway, the secretary of Dhṛtarāṣṭra could see what was going on in the battlefield, and he was in the palace, telling this to Mahārāja Dhrtarāṣṭra, who was blind. Now, the conclusion made by Sañjaya was that Kṛṣṇa is the Supreme Personality of Godhead.

When the *yoga* performance is described, it is said that Kṛṣṇa's name is *yogeśvara.* No one can be a better *yogī* than the master of *yoga,* and Kṛṣṇa is the master. There are many different types of *yoga. Yoga* means the system, and *yogī* means the person who practices that system. The object of *yoga,* the ultimate goal, is to understand Kṛṣṇa. Therefore, Kṛṣṇa consciousness means to practice the topmost type of *yoga.*

This topmost *yoga* system was described by Kṛṣṇa in the *Gītā* to His most intimate friend, Arjuna. In the beginning, the Lord said that this system can be practiced only by a person who has developed attachment for it. This Kṛṣṇa conscious *yoga* system cannot be practiced by an ordinary man who has no attachment for Kṛṣṇa, for it is a different system, and the topmost—*bhakti-yoga.*

There are five types of direct attachment, and there are seven types of indirect attachment. Indirect attachment is not *bhakti.* Direct attachment is called *bhakti.* If you are attached to Kṛṣṇa by the direct method, it is called devotional service, and if you are attached to Kṛṣṇa by an indirect method, it is not devotional service. But that is also attachment. King Kaṁsa, for example, was the maternal uncle of Kṛṣṇa; and there was a warning that Kaṁsa would be killed by one of his sister's sons. So he became very anxious about the sons of his sister, and he decided to kill his sister. Devaki, Kṛṣṇa's mother, was saved by her husband, Vasudeva, who made a compromise and proposed to his brother-in-law as follows: "You are afraid of the son of your sister. So your sister herself is not going to kill you." He requested, "Don't kill your sister. Save her, and I promise that all the sons born of her will be brought to you, and if you like you can kill them."

Vasudeva did this in order that his poor wife might

be saved. And Vasudeva thought, "When Devakī's son is born, Kaṁsa may have a change of heart." But Kaṁsa was such a great demon that he killed all the sons of Devakī. It was told that the eighth son of the sister would kill him. So, when Kṛṣṇa was in the womb of His mother, Kaṁsa was always thinking of Kṛṣṇa. You may say that he was not Kṛṣṇa conscious, but actually he was. Not directly, not for love's sake, but as an enemy. He was Kṛṣṇa conscious as an enemy. So, that is not devotional service. One in devotional service is Kṛṣṇa conscious as Kṛṣṇa's friend, Kṛṣṇa's servant, His parent, or His lover.

You may want Kṛṣṇa as your lover, or as your son; you may want Kṛṣṇa as your friend, you may want Kṛṣṇa as your master, you may want Kṛṣṇa as the Supreme Sublime. These five different kinds of direct relationships with Kṛṣṇa are called devotion, or *bhakti.* They entail no material profit.

The concept of accepting God as a son is superior to the concept of accepting God as a father. There is a distinction. The relationship between father and son is that the son wants to take something from the father. The father's relationship with the son is that the father always wants to give something to the son. Therefore, the relationship with God or Kṛṣṇa as son is better than the relationship with Kṛṣṇa by one who thinks, "If I accept God as my father, then my business will be to ask for my necessities from the father." But, if I become the father of Kṛṣṇa, then from the very beginning of His childhood, my business will be to serve Him. The father is the parent of the child from the very beginning of his birth; therefore the concept of this relationship of Vasudeva and Devakī is sublime.

Kṛṣṇa's foster mother, Yaśodā, is thinking, "If I do not feed Kṛṣṇa sumptuously, He will die." She forgets that Kṛṣṇa is the Supreme Lord, that He is sustaining the three worlds. She forgets that only one Lord is supplying the necessities of all the living entities. This same Personality of Godhead has become the son of Yaśodā, and she is thinking, "If I do not feed Him nicely, He will die." This is love. She has forgotten that it is the Supreme Personality of Godhead who has appeared before her as a little child.

This relationship of attachment is very sublime. It requires time to understand, but there is a position where, instead of asking, "O God, please give us our daily bread," you can instead think that God will die if you do not supply bread to Him. This is the ecstasy of extreme love. There is such a relationship between Kṛṣṇa and His devotee Rādhārāṇī, the greatest devotee, the greatest lover of Kṛṣṇa. Mother Yaśodā is His lover as a parent; Sudāmā is His lover as a friend; Arjuna also as a friend–there are millions and billions of different kinds of direct devotees of Kṛṣṇa.

So the *yoga* systems as described here lead to *bhakti-yoga,* and *bhakti-yoga* can be practiced by persons who have developed attachment to Kṛṣṇa. Others cannot practice it. And, if anyone is able to develop that attachment, the relationship will be that he will understand God, Kṛṣṇa, perfectly. However we may try to understand God by our different theories or speculations, it is still a difficult job. We may say that we have understood God, but it is not possible to understand Him as He is, because we have limited senses, and He is unlimited.

It is said in the *Śrīmad-Bhāgavatam* that our senses are imperfect, all of them. We cannot understand even the material world perfectly. You have seen so many planets and stars in the sky at night, but you do not know what they are. You do not even know what the moon planet is, though men have been trying for so many years to go there in sputniks. Even this one planet, Earth! We do not know what varieties there are even on this planet! If you go to the sea, to the sky, your perception is limited. Our knowledge is, therefore, always imperfect. On that we must agree. If we foolishly think that we have acquired all forms of knowledge and we have advanced in science, this is another foolishness. It is not possible.

And, when it is not possible to understand even the material things which we daily see with our eyes, what can we say of the spiritual world and Kṛṣṇa, the Supreme Personality of Godhead? He is the supreme spiritual form, and it is not possible to understand Him by our limited senses. Then why are we bothering so much for Kṛṣṇa consciousness, if it is not possible? If these imperfect senses cannot realize Kṛṣṇa as He is? The answer is that if you become submissive, if you develop the spiritual attitude of following Kṛṣṇa, and you are as a servant or a friend, as a parent or as a lover—if you begin to give service to the Supreme Lord then you can begin to know Him.

Your service begins with the tongue. How? By the tongue you can chant Hare Kṛṣṇa, and by the tongue you can taste Kṛṣṇa *prasādam*, spiritual food. So, the beginning of the process is very nice. You can chant Hare Kṛṣṇa, Hare Kṛṣṇa, Kṛṣṇa Kṛṣṇa, Hare Hare/ Hare Rāma, Hare Rāma, Rāma Rāma, Hare Hare—and whenever *prasādam* is offered to you by Kṛṣṇa, by His kindness, you accept it. The result will be that if you become submissive, and if you begin this service—chanting and eating *prasādam*—Kṛṣṇa will reveal Himself before you.

You can't understand Kṛṣṇa by speculation; that is not possible, because your senses are imperfect. But if you begin this process of service, then it will be possible—one day Kṛṣṇa will reveal Himself to you: "I am like this." Just as Kṛṣṇa is revealing to Arjuna. Arjuna is a devotee, and he is submissive, and he is in contact with Kṛṣṇa as a friend. Therefore Kṛṣṇa is revealing to him.

The *Bhagavad-gītā* was spoken to Arjuna, not to any Vedāntist philosophical speculator. In the beginning of the Fourth Chapter, you will note that Kṛṣṇa says, "I am speaking to you that ancient system of *yoga.*" It is stated, "unto you." Arjuna was a *kṣatriya*, a fighter. He was a householder, not even a *sannyāsī,* not a renouncer—but these are not qualifications to understand Kṛṣṇa. Suppose I say I have become a *sannyāsī* mendicant—this is not a qualification, that I can now understand Kṛṣṇa. Then what is the qualification? This: "One who has developed the service spirit, with love and devotion, can understand Me." No other. Not the big scholars and mental speculators; but a child can understand Kṛṣṇa, if he has full faith in Him. So faith and devotion qualify one.

Simply by such faith and service you will understand that Kṛṣṇa is the Supreme Personality of Godhead. Just as we are preaching Kṛṣṇa consciousness; we are not wasting your time or our time, because we are in full faith that Kṛṣṇa is the Supreme Personality of Godhead. Theoretically or practically, you should accept Kṛṣṇa as the Supreme Person. Theoretically, there is the revealed scripture. You will understand from the Vedic literature, from the great devotees in the past and in the present.

For the present, there is Lord Caitanya. Lord Caitanya is the great authority. None is greater. He was mad after Kṛṣṇa. And then, after Him, His six disciples, the *gosvāmīs,* have left us an immensely valuable literature—especially Jīva Gosvāmī. They have written volumes on Kṛṣṇa. So, under disciplic succession, we have come to this point; and if you like past history, then go back a long, long time to Vyāsadeva. He is known to have written the *Śrīmad-Bhāgavatam* and other literature on Kṛṣṇa. *Śrīmad-Bhāgavatam* is nothing but a description of Kṛṣṇa. Vyāsa is also the writer of the *Bhagavad-gītā.* The *Gītā* was spoken by Kṛṣṇa and noted down by Vyāsa, who put this *Gītā* into the *Mahābhārata.*

So Vyāsadeva accepts Kṛṣṇa as the Supreme Person. In the *Śrīmad-Bhāgavatam* he has given the description of the different incarnations; there are twenty-five of Them. And, in the conclusion, he says that the descriptions that are given of different incarnations are all parts of the representations of God. But Kṛṣṇa is the Supreme Personality of Godhead Himself. He is not part, but one hundred percent—one hundred percent God. So there is the evidence of authority.

And, practically, if we believe the *śāstras*, the scriptures, then we can see: Who can be more power ful than Kṛṣṇa? Who can be more beautiful than Kṛṣṇa? Who can be more famous than Kṛṣṇa? Kṛṣṇa appeared five thousand years ago, but His knowledge, which He gave in the form of the *Śrīmad Bhagavad-gītā,* is still worshiped. It is worshiped not only by the Hindus or the Indians, but is read all over the world. In your country there are at least fifty different editions of the *Bhagavad-gītā*, written by different men. Similarly, in England, in Germany, in France and in all other countries, you will find hundreds of editions of the *Gītā*. So, who can be more famous? There are many other evidences, if you believe in *śāstra:* Kṛṣṇa married 16,108 wives, and He provided each one of them with a big palace, and each one of them had 10 children, and from the 10 children there were many other children born. So we have the evidence of revealed Scriptures; and in the *Brahma-saṁhitā* also, Kṛṣṇa is accepted as the Supreme Personality of Godhead. This is a very old book, supposed to have been written by Brahmā, the first living being in the universe.

In that *Brahma-saṁhitā*, it is said, *īśvaraḥ paramaḥ kṛṣṇaḥ*. *Īśvara* means God. There are many gods. It is said that there are so many demigods, and there is the Supreme God. So *Brahma-saṁhitā* says, *īśvaraḥ paramaḥ kṛṣṇaḥ*—He is the God of gods. *Īśvaraḥ paramaḥ kṛṣṇaḥ,* and then: *sac-cid-ānanda-vigrahaḥ*—and His body is eternal, and full of bliss and knowledge. And next: *anādiḥ*—He has no beginning, but He is the beginning of everyone. *Anādir ādir govindaḥ. Go* means senses, *go* means cow, and *go* means land. He is the proprietor of all land, He is the proprietor of all cows, and He is the creator of all senses.

We are after sense pleasure, but our perfection of sense pleasure can be achieved only when we reciprocate our pleasure with Kṛṣṇa. Therefore, His name is Govinda, the Supreme Original Personality of Godhead.

The same Personality of Godhead personally spoke about Himself to Arjuna in the *Gītā.* How can you say that somebody, by his thinking, by speculation, can say something about God that is more important than what is being said by Kṛṣṇa Himself? It is not possible. No one can speak better than Kṛṣṇa about God, because God Himself is speaking. If you speak about yourself personally, who can say more than you? So, if you have faith, if you believe theoretically or practically in Kṛṣṇa as the Supreme Personality of Godhead, then, by the speeches that are delivered by Kṛṣṇa in the *Bhagavad-gītā,* you can understand God. There is no difficulty.

And, if you believe Kṛṣṇa, then the result will be that you can understand God—how He is working, how His energies are acting, how He is manifesting, what is this material world, what is the spiritual world, what are the living creatures, what is their relationship—so many things are to be found in God's literature.

The whole Vedic literature deals with three things: the first is your relationship with God; then, next, after you understand your relationship with God, you can act in that way. Just as a man or woman may not be related, but as soon as the relationship is established that one is husband and the other is wife, then the dealings begin.

Once they understand their relationship with God, people generally believe that God is the father, and the son's business is to ask Father for whatever he needs. But that is really a lesser relationship. If you understand God perfectly, then there are intimate relationships also. Your intimate relationship will be revealed when you are perfectly liberated. Each and every living creature has a particular relationship with God, but we have, for now, forgotten. When that relationship is revealed in the process of devotional activities, or Kṛṣṇa consciousness, you will know that that is the perfection of your life. Kṛṣṇa consciousness is a great science; it is not a sentimental speculation regarding love. It is based on scientific propositions described in the *Bhagavad-gītā,* in the *Vedas,* and in the *Brahma-saṁhitā;* and it is accepted by authorities like Lord Caitanya, Rāmānujācārya, Madhvācārya, Nārada, Asita, Vyāsa—there are so many authorities. Kṛṣṇa consciousness is not an ordinary lovemaking or moneymaking business; it is reality, and if you stick to it seriously, your life will be perfect.

Kṛṣṇa says in *Bhagavad-gītā,* "After giving up this body, one who knows Me in truth does not come back again to this material world to accept a material body." Then what happens to him? He goes to Kṛṣṇa, back home, back to Godhead. This Kṛṣṇa consciousness movement is directly giving people understanding of Kṛṣṇa. We are giving knowledge of Kṛṣṇa based on these authorized scriptures: *Bhagavad-gītā* and the *Vedas. Veda* means knowledge, and *Vedānta* means the ultimate end of knowledge. What is that end of knowledge? That is Kṛṣṇa. *Vedaiś ca sarvair aham eva vedyaḥ.* By knowing all the *Vedas,* the ultimate conclusion should be Kṛṣṇa. This conclusion comes after many, many births. After culturing knowledge for many, many births, when one actually becomes wise, then he surrenders unto Kṛṣṇa. How can he surrender? He knows that Vāsudeva, Kṛṣṇa, is everything. Whatever we see is simply a manifestation of the energy of Vāsudeva. One must be convinced on this point, and then he becomes a devotee. Kṛṣṇa therefore advises that whether you understand or not, simply surrender unto Him. What Kṛṣṇa taught in *Bhagavad-gītā,* we are also teaching, without different manufactured ideas. That is our Kṛṣṇa consciousness movement. It is open to everyone, and the process is very simple. We have our centers. If you want to take advantage of this movement, you are welcome. You will be happy.

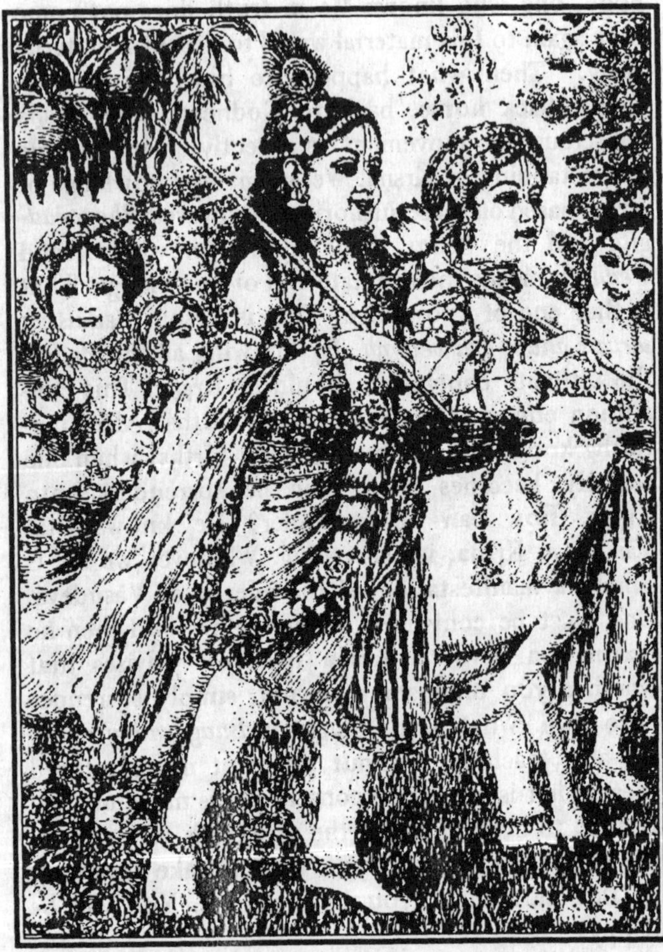

3 Beyond the Laws of Nature

In materialistic life we cannot control our senses and mind. The mind is dictating, "Enjoy your senses in this way," and we are enjoying our senses. Materialistic life means sense gratification. This sense gratification process is going on life after life. In the many varieties of life there are different standards of sense gratification. Kṛṣṇa is so kind that He has given us full liberty to gratify our senses.

We are part and parcel of Kṛṣṇa; we have small particles of all the desires of Kṛṣṇa. Our existence is a small particle of God's, just like a small particle of gold which has all the qualities of the original gold. Kṛṣṇa has the propensity for sense gratification. He is the original sense gratifier. It is stated in *Bhagavad-gītā* that Kṛṣṇa is the supreme enjoyer. Our enjoying spirit exists because it exists originally in Kṛṣṇa.

The *Vedānta-sūtra* says that everything originates from Kṛṣṇa. *Param Brahman,* or the Absolute Truth, means that from which everything is generated. Therefore, our desire for sense gratification is coming from Kṛṣṇa. Here is the perfect sense gratification—Kṛṣṇa and Rādhārāṇī. Young boys and girls are similarly trying to enjoy their senses, but where is this propensity coming from? It is coming from Kṛṣṇa. Because we are part and parcel of Kṛṣṇa, the quality of desire for sense gratification exists within us. But the difference is that we are trying to gratify our senses in the material world; therefore we are perverted. In Kṛṣṇa consciousness one gratifies his senses in association with Kṛṣṇa. Then it is perfect.

For example, if there is a nice sweetball or some nice foodstuff and the finger picks it up, it cannot enjoy. The foodstuff has to be given to the stomach, and then the finger can also enjoy. Similarly, we cannot gratify our senses directly. But when we join with Kṛṣṇa, when Kṛṣṇa enjoys, then we can enjoy. That is our position. The finger cannot eat anything independently; it cannot enjoy the nice sweetball. The finger can pick it up and put it in the stomach, and when the stomach enjoys, then the finger enjoys.

We have to purify the propensity of material sense gratification. That is Kṛṣṇa consciousness. For Kṛṣṇa consciousness we have to be purified. What is that purification? We cannot enjoy anything directly, so we have to enjoy through Kṛṣṇa. For example, we take *prasādam*. The nice *prasādam*, the foodstuff that is prepared, is not taken directly—we take it through Kṛṣṇa. First of all, we offer to Kṛṣṇa, and then we take it.

What is the difficulty? There is no difficulty, but you become purified. The eating process is the same, but if you eat directly then you become materialistically encumbered. If you offer to Kṛṣṇa, however, and then take it, then you become freed from all contamination of material life. That is stated in *Bhagavad-gītā*. Devotees take *prasādam* after offering it to Kṛṣṇa. That is called sacrifice. Whatever you offer to Kṛṣṇa or Viṣṇu is called sacrifice. Whatever we do here, within this material world, is some sort of sinful activity, even if we do not know it. Killing is sinful activity, even if we do not kill willingly. When you walk down the street you are killing many animals. Whenever you drink water, you are also killing. Below a water pot there are many ants and microbes that are being killed. Whenever you light a fire, there are many small microbes that also burn in the fire. When you grind spices with a mortar and pestle, many small microbes are killed.

We are responsible for this. Willingly or unwillingly, we are becoming entangled in many sinful activities. Therefore, *Bhagavad-gītā* says that if you take the remnants of foodstuff after offering sacrifice, you become freed from all contamination. Otherwise, one who cooks to eat personally without offering to Kṛṣṇa is simply eating sinful reactions. This is our position. Therefore, it is stated that because people generally cannot control their senses, they engage in the materialistic way of life in which repeated birth and death in different species takes place.

I do not know what is my next life, but the next life will come. Before us there are many species of life; I can take birth in any one of them. I can become a demigod, I can become a cat, I can become a dog, I can become Brahmā–there are so many forms of life. In the next life I shall have to accept one of these forms, even if I do not want to. Suppose someone asks, "In your next life would you like to take the form of a dog or a hog?" I would not like it. But the law of nature says that after giving up this body, when I am not existing in this body any more, I will have to accept another body according to my *karma*. That is in the hands of nature. It is arranged by superior supervision. You cannot order, "Give me the body of Brahmā, give me the body of Indra or a king or something exalted." That is not in your hands or in my hands; that will be judged by the superior agency of God, Kṛṣṇa, and you will be given a body. Therefore, it is our duty to prepare a body which will help us go back to Kṛṣṇa. That is Kṛṣṇa consciousness.

Prahlāda Mahārāja, a great authority, says that one must take instruction from others. One must take instruction from a *guru,* a spiritual master. One should not take instruction from anyone unless one accepts him as a *guru.* But even one who has a nice *guru* cannot remain Kṛṣṇa conscious if he is determined to remain in this material world. If my determination is to remain in this material world to enjoy material life, then for me Kṛṣṇa consciousness is impossible.

Everyone in the material world is engaged in all kinds of political, philanthropic and humanitarian activities to make material life happy and prosperous, but this is not possible. One should understand that in the material world, however one may try to make adjustments, he cannot be happy. To cite an example I have given many times, if you take a fish out of water, you can give it a very comfortable velvet bedstead, but still the fish cannot be happy; it will die. Because the fish is an animal of the water, it cannot be happy without water. Similarly, we are all spirit soul; unless we are in spiritual life or in the spiritual world, we cannot be happy. That is our position.

Everyone is trying for that spiritual realization. But we do not know. Therefore, we are trying to be happy here, in material conditions. We are becoming frustrated and confused. Therefore, we have to withdraw this understanding that we shall be very happy by making adjustments to this material world. Then Kṛṣṇa consciousness will be effective.

The boys and girls who are our students have been very scornful of the materialistic way of life. Their fathers and guardians are not poor. There is no scarcity of food or material enjoyments. Why are they being frustrated? You may say that because India is poverty-stricken the people are frustrated, but why have American boys and girls been frustrated? That is the proof that the materialistic way of life cannot make you happy. You may go on for some time trying to become happy, but happiness will never come from materialistic life.That is a fact. Those who are trying to be happy by making material adjustments cannot take to Kṛṣṇa consciousness. Frustration and confusion with materialistic life is the qualification to come to Kṛṣṇa consciousness. These boys and girls have a good qualification; they are coming to Kṛṣṇa consciousness. There is a verse in *Śrīmad-Bhāgavatam* which states that sometimes to show special favor to His devotees Kṛṣṇa takes away all one's material opulence. For example, the Pāṇḍavas were bereft of their kingdom, although Kṛṣṇa was present there. Kṛṣṇa was present as their friend, and still they were bereft of their kingdom. They lost their property, their wife was insulted, and they were driven away to the forest.

This question was posed by Yudhiṣṭhira Mahārāja to Kṛṣṇa. "How is it," he inquired indirectly, "that

You are our friend and that we are put into such difficulty?" Kṛṣṇa replied to Yudhiṣṭhira Mahārāja, "This is My special favor." Sometimes we cannot understand the special favor of Kṛṣṇa.

So this frustration of the American and English boys with the materialistic way of life is a good sign for accepting Kṛṣṇa consciousness. Of course, one does not need to become poor to take to Kṛṣṇa consciousness. But if anyone has the desire to become spiritually advanced while at the same time enjoying material life, that is not possible. These are two contradictory aspirations. One must become determined to be happy in spiritual life. That is real happiness.

This human form is especially meant for coming to that standard of spiritual life by *tapasya,* by voluntarily rejecting the materialistic way of life. In the history of India there were many great kings like Bharat Mahārāja who even at a very young age practiced *tapasya.* Bharat Mahārāja at the age of only twenty-four years left his young wife, young children and the whole empire Bhāratavarṣa and went to the forest for meditation. There are many such instances. Prahlāda Mahārāja was questioned by his father, Hiraṇyakaśipu, "Who has taught you this Kṛṣṇa consciousness?" A king's son does not mix with anyone else; he simply takes lessons from the appointed teachers. How is it then that this boy, who was only five years old, was so Kṛṣṇa conscious? His father was surprised, so he asked him, "How have you taken to Kṛṣṇa consciousness?" The answer was, "My dear father, Kṛṣṇa consciousness cannot be achieved by a person like you, whose job is always simply to enjoy this material world." *Hiraṇya* means gold, and *kaśipu* means softly cushioned bed.

Materialistic life is spent chewing the chewed. Take, for instance, a father. A father knows that he has responsibilities, so he works hard to maintain his family. It is very difficult to keep the high standard of living in this age, so one must work very hard and engage one's son in the same way. In spite of very bad experience with materialistic life, still one engages his son in the same way. This happens again and again, so it is like chewing chewed things. Once I have chewed sugar cane and taken its juice, it is thrown out in the street, and if someone wants to taste it to see how sweet it is, he is chewing the chewed. Similarly, we don't have very good experience with this materialistic life, this hard struggle for life, but human beings, as it is stated in the *Śrīmad-Bhāgavatam,* are born of the quality of passion. There are three qualities in the material world: goodness, passion and ignorance. Because people are in the mode of passion, they love to work very hard. That hard work is considered happiness. In London you will see everyone engaged in hard work. In the morning, all the buses and trucks travel with great speed, and people go to the office or factory from morning until late at night. They work hard, and it is called advancement of civilization. Some of them are frustrated; they don't want it. There will be frustration—after all, it is hard work. Hogs, too, are working hard day and night, thinking, "Where is stool? Where is stool?" That is their business. Therefore, in one sense this kind of civilization is a hog and dog civilization. It is not human civilization. Human civilization means sobriety. One should be inquisitive. A human being should be inquisitive to know these things: Who am I? Why am I put into this condition of working very hard to get only a few grains? Why am I in this uncomfortable situation? Where did I come from? Where do I have to go? The *Vedānta-sūtra* begins by stating that a human being should be inquisitive to know who he is, where he comes from, and where he has to go. Kṛṣṇa consciousness is for those who have come to detest this material world. They are good candidates for developing Kṛṣṇa consciousness. They will inquire why these men are working so hard and what their goal in life is.

That is answered in *Śrīmad-Bhāgavatam.* People are working so hard because they do not actually know what the goal of life is. Everyone says that he is looking after his self-interest, but he does not know what his self-interest is. *Na te viduḥ svārtha-gatiṁ hi viṣṇu.* He should know that his real self-interest is to make progress toward Viṣṇu, the Supreme Personality of Godhead. They do not know this. Why don't they know it? Because they have hopes which are very difficult to fulfill. I may hope for something which is possible; that is good. But if I hope for something which is never possible, that is hope which will never be fulfilled.

We are a composition of the external and internal energies of God. The gross external energy is this gross material body, and the subtle external energy is the mind, ego and intelligence. Behind both energies—the gross external energy and the subtle external energy—is the soul, the internal energy. This body is made of earth, water, fire, air and ether. This is called gross external energy, and there is also a subtle external energy of mind, intelligence and false ego. And behind that, the soul is there.

I am the proprietor of this body. Just as one is covered by a shirt and coat which are external to his real body, similarly we are covered by this gross body made up of earth, water, fire, air and ether, which is the gross external energy of God, or Kṛṣṇa, and the mind, ego and intelligence, which are subtle. Thus we are covered.

I may think that simply by having a nice shirt and coat I can be happy, but is it possible? Unless you eat nicely, unless you sleep nicely, unless you have your sense gratification, will you be happy simply by putting on a costly shirt and coat? No. That is not possible. We want to be happy by adjustment of this external energy. That cannot be. You are spirit soul—you must have spiritual food, you must have a spiritual life, and then you can be happy. As you cannot be happy simply by having a nice shirt and coat, similarly simply by the materialistic way of life you cannot be happy. There is gross matter and subtle matter. Gross matter includes high skyscraper buildings, machines, factories, nice roads, good cars, etc. Subtle matter includes nice songs, poetry, philosophy, etc. People are trying to be happy with this gross and subtle material existence. That cannot be.

Why have people accepted this sort of civilization? Because they are led by blind leaders. We are conducting this Kṛṣṇa consciousness movement, and very few are interested. But suppose we advertise some falsehood—"If you follow this path, within six months you will become God, and you will be all-powerful." Many people would come. This is actually one blind man leading other blind men. Suppose one blind man says, "All right, come, follow me. I shall help you crossing this busy Mulberry Street." He is blind, and the followers are also blind. The result will be that they will be hit by some car or truck and they will all die.

We do not know that we are bound by the stringent laws of material nature. How can we become free from this material bondage? We have to take instruction from those who are not blind, whose eyes are opened and who are liberated from this material bondage. One must take instruction from such persons, and then he will understand his self-interest. Otherwise, if one who is blind takes instruction from a blind man, it will not be possible for him to be liberated from material bondage.

What is self-interest? What is the interest of a child when it is crying? It is searching after the mother's breast. Anyone who knows this immediately brings the child to its mother—"Take care of your child; he is crying." The mother takes him to her breast, and the child is immediately happy. The child cannot express what he wants, so he simply cries. But one who knows what he is crying for helps him, and the child becomes happy. Similarly, because we are part and parcel of Kṛṣṇa, the Supreme Lord, the Supreme Personality of Godhead, we are actually crying for Kṛṣṇa. But these false leaders, these blind leaders who do not know, are giving stone instead of bread.

How can one be happy? I have already explained the gross external energy and the subtle external energy. Those who are interested in this gross and subtle external energy will never have their ambition of life fulfilled. One who is interested in Viṣṇu and in showing the path of Viṣṇu is the real friend. One who is giving Kṛṣṇa consciousness is the real friend of the world. No others can give happiness to human society. That is the explanation given by Prahlāda Mahārāja.

You cannot manufacture a process of happiness by tackling this material energy. That is not possible because the material energy is not under your control. It is controlled by the Supreme. How can you overpower the material energy? It is not possible. That is explained in *Bhagavad-gītā.* It is not possible to overcome the stringent laws of material nature. Kṛṣṇa says, "It is My energy; I am the controller. But one can surrender unto Me."

All the material activities of the cosmic manifestation are going on just to bring the rebellious souls back to Godhead. That is the situation. *Māyā's* stringent laws are there. Why? What is the purpose of the police force or the military force? The purpose is to keep the citizens obedient to the state. If a citizen is disobedient to the state law, he is immediately put into police custody. Similarly, anyone who has rebelled against the superiority of God is put under the stringent laws of material nature, and he must suffer. That is the position. Therefore, his self-interest is to seek out the Supreme Personality of Godhead and surrender unto Him. That will make him happy. Otherwise, if he simply tries to accept material things and become happy, that is not possible.

Prahlāda Mahārāja gives a hint as to how one can seek out the path of Viṣṇu, or Kṛṣṇa consciousness. He says that we have created so many unnecessary things and become entangled by them. In the beginning of *Śrīmad-Bhāgavatam* it is stated that we should desire to get out of this unnecessary trouble and to be free from the problems which are created. This morning I saw a picture of Berlin which was sent by one of my disciples. I have been to Berlin and to Moscow, and both are very nice cities. Berlin is a very nice city and London is also a very nice city, but why do the people engage in fighting and bombing every other city? Why has this happened? Because they have lost their interest in Viṣṇu, God. Therefore, they are thinking, "You are my enemy; I am your enemy," and they fight like cats and dogs. But as soon as we come to the Viṣṇu understanding, the Kṛṣṇa understanding, these advanced cities, these advanced civilizations, can be maintained very nicely. You'll be happy, you'll eat nicely, dance nicely, live nicely and go back home, back to Godhead. Enjoy this life and the next life. That is our request.

Everyone should take the Kṛṣṇa consciousness movement seriously and try to understand it seriously. It is authorized on the Vedic principle; it is not something manufactured or unauthorized. We are opening centers in different parts of the world to give an opportunity for people to understand their real interest: Viṣṇu, Kṛṣṇa. That is our mission. Kindly help us and join us.

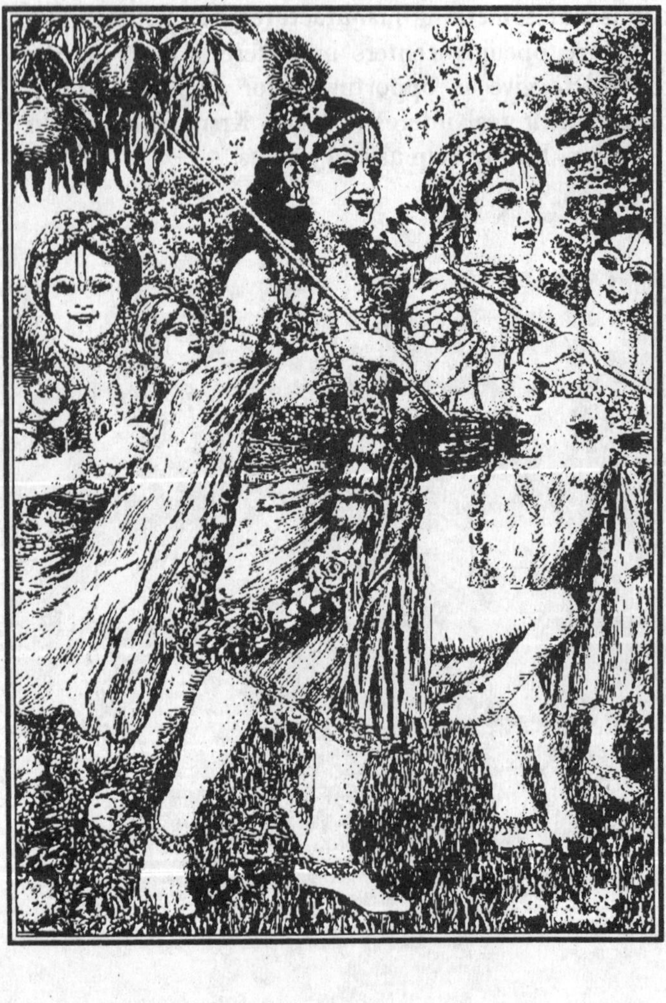

4

The Goal of Yoga

In the *Bhagavad-gītā*, the Sanskrit word *mām* is frequently used. This word means "unto me." Kṛṣṇa, the Supreme Personality of Godhead, says, "unto Me"—Kṛṣṇa. We cannot interpret this in a different way. When I say, "Bring me a glass of water," it means that I am the person in want of the glass of water, and if you supply to me and not to others, then it is right. When Kṛṣṇa says, "unto Me," that means Kṛṣṇa. But philosophers are still interpreting—they say "unto something else." Even grammatically this is wrong.

One who has developed attachment to Kṛṣṇa is Kṛṣṇa conscious. They say if you have attachment for your lover you always think of her. That is lover consciousness. It is natural. It is stated that a woman who has another lover besides her husband shows herself very attentive to her household duties, but is always thinking, "When shall my lover and I meet in the night?" This is an example. It is possible, in spite of our false engagement, if we love somebody, to think of him always. If materially it is possible, why not spiritually? That is the whole teaching of the *Bhagavad-gītā*.

In the *Gītā,* Kṛṣṇa says to Arjuna, "As a fighter, you have to fight. You cannot step away from the fighting. It is your duty." Nowadays I have practical experience that the draft board of your country is calling for boys to join the army, but they are not willing. They are not willing because they are not trained as *kṣatriyas,* warriors. They are trained as *śūdras,* laborers. Therefore the caste system is very scientific. A section of people should be trained as *brāhmaṇas,* men of knowledge. Those who are intelligent enough in the society should be picked and trained in higher philosophical science. And those who are less intelligent than the *brāhmaṇas* should be given military training. We require everything in society—not only military men. How can everyone be a military man? Because they are sending *śūdras,* ordinary workers, to Vietnam, these are unnecessarily being killed. Any country which is very proud of scientific advancement, and yet does not know how to organize its society, is a fool's society.

In the *Bhagavad-gītā* Kṛṣṇa says that there are four divisions of society, *brāhmaṇa, kṣatriya, vaiśya* and *śūdra.* That is natural. Some are inclined toward spiritual advancement, and these are the *brāhmaṇas.* Now we are training boys who are spiritually inclined and they are unnecessarily being forced into military service. The foolish have no knowledge that some boy is being trained up in higher science. Why should he be destroyed when he is being perfected? The intellectual persons, those boys who have brahminical qualifications, are being restrained in *brahmacarya* student life: they don't take to meat-eating, they don't take part in illicit sex. They are being trained as complete *brāhmaṇas,* the highest intellectuals, the most purified persons in society. If there is one *brāhmaṇa* in a whole family, then the whole family—the whole society—becomes sanctified. But today they have no knowledge of how to train a *brāhmaṇa,* or how to train a *kṣatriya.* In the other fields of action, in the work of *śūdras* and *vaiśyas* there is nice training. If anyone wants to be a businessman, there are colleges or technological schools. That's very nice. But why should everyone be dragged into technology? Just as in your body: for proper maintenance we require the head, the arms, the belly and the legs. All these parts of the body are required. You cannot say, "We do not require the head." That is nonsense—we require everything. Suppose there is a body without a head—it is a dead body. If the body is now intact, but there is no head, it is called a dead body. The head is considered to be the intellectual part of the body. Similarly, if there is no *brāhmaṇa* in the society, it is a dead body. If there is no spiritual man in the society, it is a dead society.

Therefore, Kṛṣṇa says, "I have created the four divisions of society, according to quality and work." If someone is working as a *brahmacārī-brāhmaṇa* and has acquired the quality of understanding Kṛṣṇa, the Supreme Lord, then why should he be called for army action? The arm of the body is the *kṣatriya.* Of course that is required; to protect the society, to protect the country, a military arrangement should be there. No one will disapprove. But not the *brāhmaṇas.* It is putting a race horse before the work cart. A race horse is required for different purposes. The other beasts of burden—asses, mules and oxen—are required for pulling carts.

I say this frankly—everyone may read it—that any society where there are no spiritual persons or Kṛṣṇa consciousness is a rascal society, because it has no head. Where there is a headless man, there is a dead body. And if there is no brain, there is no head; if the brain is not working properly then he is a madman; if he has no head at all, then he is a dead man.

Do you think that in a dead society or a mad society there can be any peace? No. If the society is full of madmen, then where is the question of peace? Therefore, Kṛṣṇa consciousness is the most important study in present-day society. The men who are leading the society, the President and the Secretary of Defense, should have the intelligence to understand this science of the soul.

The other day when coming to your country I met a secretary of the Japanese government in Tokyo. I wanted to explain to him that he should cooperate with this movement, but he said, "Oh, we cannot cooperate with any religious movement." He is one of the chief secretaries of the government, and he is such a fool. He is taking this movement as a religious movement, just as we have so many sentimental religions. But this is not sentimental. This is the necessity of society: a class of men should be Kṛṣṇa conscious. Otherwise the society is doomed; it is going to hell. And, when such rascals are at the head of the government, how can there be peace? How can you expect peace in a dog's society? The dogs are by nature howling—"Woof! Woof! Woof!"—as soon as they see other dogs. So do you mean to say there will be peace if you turn human society into dog society, into cat society, into tiger society? The tiger is very powerful; he can kill many other animals. But does that mean he is a very important animal? No, he has no use in society. And now we are very powerful, and we have good weapons to fight with, and we can kill many people. But these are no qualifications for good men or a good society.

We are not meant to manufacture a society of monkeys or tigers or asses—or rascals who work very hard. Do you mean to say a society of asses will derive any benefit from life? No.

For those who have developed an attraction to Kṛṣṇa, attachment can be developed. Before my coming to the West, there was no movement like this Kṛṣṇa consciousness, but now it is developing. Kṛṣṇa was not born in your country; you do not accept Kṛṣṇa as your religious God. But Kṛṣṇa is so attractive that although you are a foreigner, you are not foreign. To Kṛṣṇa you are not a foreigner. He claims everybody. We make Him foreign, but this is our foolishness.

In the *Gītā* Kṛṣṇa says, "My dear Arjuna, there are many different forms and different species of life undoubtedly. But I am their father." Just see how Kṛṣṇa is universal. He is claiming not only human society, but animal society, bird society, beast society—everyone. He says, "I am the father." So how can Kṛṣṇa be foreign? It is a mental concoction. They say Kṛṣṇa is Indian or Kṛṣṇa is worshiped by the Hindus and therefore He is one of the Hindu Gods; and they think that Kṛṣṇa is saying, "Yes, I am the Hindu God. Yes, I am Indian." But He is like the sun. Why American sun or Indian? Nothing is American or Indian; that is all artificial.

"This planet belongs to the humans, that's all." This is your communism. This present communism is defective because the Russians say that Russia is for the Russians or China is for the Chinese. Why not for others? Just think in terms of human communism! Why human communism? Living being communism! If you take this world as belonging to human society, that is defective. It belongs to everyone! It belongs to the tree community; it belongs to the beast community. They also have a right to live. Why should you cut the trees? Why should you send the bulls to the slaughterhouse? This is injustice. How can you gain justice by yourself doing injustice? We have no Kṛṣṇa consciousness. We do not know that Kṛṣṇa is our original father and that we are all His sons. The tree is my brother, the ant is my brother, the bull is my brother. The American is my brother, the Indian is my brother, the Chinese is my brother. Therefore, we have to develop Kṛṣṇa consciousness. We talk all this nonsense of universal brotherhood and United Nations—all nonsense. Either you acknowledge the Father, or else you have no idea of how to realize brotherhood or humanity. Therefore, they are talking for years and years. They are the same fools. Can't you see the U.N.? They have headquarters in New York. They are simply talking nonsense, that's all. That is their business. So unless there is full Kṛṣṇa consciousness, there cannot be any improvement of the world condition.

Kṛṣṇa says that you have to develop your attachment for Him. Begin at the beginning, but you can do it; it is not artificial. I have a few sincere students here, just developing; they are not complete, but they are developing Kṛṣṇa-attachment. Otherwise, why should they waste their time chanting Hare Kṛṣṇa? They are doing it, and it can be done. You can develop love for anything if you try for it. But Kṛṣṇa development is very natural. Because Kṛṣṇa is not a thing belonging to a particular type of religion or sect. Kṛṣṇa claims, "I belong to everyone." Therefore originally, we are all connected with Kṛṣṇa; but we have simply forgotten. This process of chanting is to evoke your remembrance of Kṛṣṇa. It is not that we are inducting something artificially into you. No, Kṛṣṇa is already connected with you, but you have forgotten. And we are trying to give you the process for reviving your original consciousness. So you can come to our temple; that is the beginning. You can see Kṛṣṇa or Kṛṣṇa's devotees, and you can chant Hare Kṛṣṇa.

Kṛṣṇa is not different from His name because He is absolute. He is nondifferent from His words. The name Kṛṣṇa and the person Kṛṣṇa are not different. Because everything is Kṛṣṇa.

Oneness, the philosophy of monism or pantheism, is imperfect. When that oneness comes in understanding Kṛṣṇa, that is perfection. If Kṛṣṇa is the Supreme Absolute Truth from whom everything is emanating, then everything is Kṛṣṇa. Just as you have a gold mine and are preparing so many golden utensils and ornaments and many other things. But they are all gold because the original is gold. So you may name it "earring," but you have to add "gold"—golden earring. You may name it "necklace," but it is gold, because originally it came from the goldmine. Similarly, originally, everything is coming from Kṛṣṇa.

If He is Supreme, the Absolute Truth, then nothing is different from Him. Just as, whether you say earring or necklace or bangle or wristwatch, these are all made of gold, and so they are gold. But, at the same time, you cannot say that this is all gold—you must say, "This is a gold necklace. This is a gold earring." The *māyāvādī,* or impersonalist, will say that everything is *Brahman.* But "everything is *Brahman*" is not right.

This is very nicely explained in the *Gītā,* in the Thirteenth Chapter: "I am expanded all over. That is My impersonal feature." Kṛṣṇa is everywhere in His impersonal feature, but still He is a person. The *māyāvādī* philosopher thinks that if Kṛṣṇa has become everything, then where is the possibility of Kṛṣṇa here, apart? This is complete rascaldom because it is thinking in a material way. There is no spiritual knowledge.

In the material way, suppose you take a piece of paper and tear it into particles and throw it all over. The original paper has no existence. This is material. But we get information from the *Vedas* that the Absolute Truth is so perfect that if you take away the whole, still the whole remains. One minus one equals one. The material way of thinking is one minus one equals zero; but spiritually it is not like that. Spiritually, one minus one equals one, and one plus one equals one also.

Kṛṣṇa is everything. The *māyāvādīs,* the impersonalists, see our Deities here and say, "Oh, they have installed some wooden forms, and they are worshiping them as God." But one who knows Kṛṣṇa science understands that Kṛṣṇa is everything and therefore can appear in everything. With electricity, the current is everywhere along the line, so wherever you touch you will feel it. Similarly, the Kṛṣṇa current in His impersonal form is everywhere, and it is the technician who knows how to use the force. Before we have a phone installed, we have a telephone conversation, and we simply inform the person, before we even talk money, that he should come immediately to find out where the connection can be made. And he comes out and does his work; and we do not notice, because he knows the technique. So, one must know how to connect with Kṛṣṇa. Kṛṣṇa is everywhere—this is Kṛṣṇa consciousness. But one must know how he can derive Kṛṣṇa from the features of Kṛṣṇa's form in wood or iron or metal.

You have to learn how to contact Kṛṣṇa everywhere in everything. That is explained in the system of *yoga.* Kṛṣṇa consciousness is also *yoga,* the perfect *yoga,* the highest of all yogic systems. A *yogī* may come, and we can challenge him, saying that this is the topmost *yoga* system, though at the same time it is very simple. You don't have to exercise your body over a period of weeks before you feel some power. But in Kṛṣṇa consciousness you won't feel tired. All of our students are simply anxious to be overloaded with work in Kṛṣṇa consciousness. "Prabhupāda, what can I do?" And they are actually doing it. In the material world, if you work for some time you'll feel weak.

Of course, I am not exercising myself. I am an old man of seventy-two years. I was ill, I went back to India; but I want to work. Actually, I could retire from all these activities, but as far as I can, I want to work; I want to learn day and night. At night I will work with the dictaphone, and I am sorry if I cannot work. This is Kṛṣṇa consciousness. One must be very anxious to work. It is not an idle society. No, we have sufficient engagements: editing papers, selling papers.

Simply find out how Kṛṣṇa conscious you can be. If you want to be really at peace, if you want to be happy, then develop Kṛṣṇa consciousness. And the beginning is to develop attachment for Kṛṣṇa. The process which we have prescribed is chanting and dancing before the Deities, and offering *prasādam*, spiritual food. This will make you more Kṛṣṇa conscious.

The *yoga* system as it is described in the *Bhagavad-gītā* is different from the bogus *yoga* system which is going on in the West these days. The *yoga* systems which have been introduced into the West by so-called *yogīs* are not bona fide. *Yoga* is difficult: the first thing is to control the senses. That is the position of the *yogī:* he is not allowed to indulge in sex life. If you indulge in intoxication, if you indulge in meat-eating, and if you indulge in gambling and sporting—

all nonsense—you cannot at the same time become a *yogī*. I was astonished when a *yogī* came here, having advertised in India that you can be a *yogī* even though you may be addicted to drinking. This is not the *yoga* system. This is not standard. You can call it *yoga*, but it is not the standard *yoga* system.

The *yoga* system is especially difficult for this age. In the *Śrīmad-Bhāgavatam* we understand that *yoga* means to concentrate one's attention on the Superself, Viṣṇu. He is situated in your heart. And, in order to concentrate your attention, you have to control the senses. The senses are working just like infuriated horses. If you cannot control the horses of your carriage, it will be dangerous. Just imagine that you are seated in a carriage and your horses are so furious that they are dragging you to hell. Then what is your position? The *yoga* system means to control these senses. The senses are also compared to serpents: The serpent does not know who is its friend and who is its enemy. It bites anyone. And, as soon as the serpent bites, the result is death. Similarly, if the uncontrolled senses work in their own way, then you should know that you are in a dangerous position.

It has been said that when one becomes too sensual, he loses his temper, he loses his identity, he forgets himself. Infuriated by the senses, a man will attack even his children, even his daughter. Therefore, for those who are advancing in spiritual life—not only for them but for everyone—the *śāstras*, scriptures, say that you should not sit in a secluded place even with your mother, even with your daughter or your sister. Why? Because the senses are so strong that if they become infuriated, you will forget whether she's mother, sister, or daughter.

You may say that this may be true only for some foolish persons, but *śāstra* says no—you should not sit in a secluded place even with your mother, sister or daughter, because the senses are so strong that even though you may be very moral, you may still be attracted by sex.

Our position in this world, our suffering in this world, is due to the body. This body is the cause of all miseries, and the ultimate goal of life should be to get out of this material body and be situated in the spiritual body. This is a foreign atmosphere. The soul is free spiritually, but it has been conditioned by this material atmosphere. And the body is of this matter.

A human being is fit to inquire as to whether he is this body or something else. This can be understood very easily. I am not this body, because at the time of death the body remains—although everyone cries, "Oh, the poor man is gone!" The man is lying there. Why do you say he is gone? He is lying there! At that time, we can come to our senses: the body is not the man. The real man is gone. The childhood body is changed to the youthful body, and the childhood body is gone. Similarly, when the boyhood body is gone, you'll have to accept a body like mine, an old man's body. The body is changing. Not only year after year, but at every second the body is changing. Still, you are situated there. This is very simple to understand. And because the body is there, we are suffering. Everyone is trying to get out of suffering, in any field of action; in the economic field, in the political field, or any field of activity, social or national, everyone is trying to get out of misery. There is no other activity. Either nationally or socially, individually or collectively, we are all suffering; and this suffering is due to the body.

Yoga means to inquire. What am I? If I am not this body, then what am I? I am pure soul. Now, if my bodily activities or sensual activities are incorrect, I will not be able to understand myself—what I am—and the *Bhagavad-gītā* says that we are all grand fools. Why fools? Since we have this body, we are fools. If somebody invites you to come to his apartment but you know it is full of danger, do you think you would like to go there? "Oh no," you will say, "I am not going there. If it is full of danger, why shall I go?" Similarly, don't you think that the body is full of danger? Then, why are you going there, taking repeated birth? When you are flying in a plane, you are always fearful that there may be a crash. And what is this crashing? It is due to the body. The soul cannot be affected by crashes. But you are always afraid.

The soul is ever-existing, and the body will not exist. And because you are existing and the soul has accepted the nonexisting body, therefore you suffer.

The problem, then, is how to get out, just as you try to get out of a fever. The fevered condition is not your permanent life. Permanent life is enjoyment, but due to the fever you cannot enjoy life. When you are sick you cannot go out; you have to rest and take so many medicines and formulas. But we don't want that—"Why should I be a sick person?" But you are diseased. Similarly, we should always know that this bodily conditional stage of the pure soul is a diseased condition. And anyone who does not know that he is suffering from disease is a fool. He is Fool Number One.

The *śāstra* says, everyone is born a fool: because he has this body, therefore he was born a fool. No being, either American or Indian, cat or dog, is free from this. You have come to disease, that's all. If you feel, "I am an American," that is a kind of disease; if you feel, "I am an Indian," that is also a disease; if you feel, "I am a cat," that is a disease. You are not a cat, you are not a dog, you are not Indian, you are not fair, you are not black. You are your soul—that is your identity! And one who does not understand this truth, that "I am pure soul," is defeated in all his activities.

Lord Jesus Christ taught like that: If you lose your soul and gain the whole world, what do you gain? People do not know what they are, and yet they work just like madmen. Just see, all these people are working, and they are madmen. They are not Americans or Indians, Germans or Japanese. They are nothing of the kind. They have been given a chance to come to this naughty place, this Earth; and so, being born in a particular place, they have a particular kind of body—and they are mad after it.

The *Bhagavad-gītā* says that just as our outer garments are changed, so this body is changed. *Yoga* means the process of getting out of this material embodiment. Just as you are repeating changes of dress, so you are repeating birth and death, and this is the cause of your miseries. If you do not understand this, then all your activities end in defeat.

Yoga means to get out of this embodiment, and it means to know oneself. This body is born of the parents. Similarly, as pure soul, you are also the source of its birth. We do not mean birth beginning historically from a certain day and ending on a certain day. No; the soul is not like that–it has no beginning, and it has no end. But in the *Bhagavad-gītā* it is said that the soul is part and parcel of God. God is eternal, God is full of joy and bliss. The position of the Absolute Person, the Godhead, is that He is full of bliss, eternal, and full of knowledge. And, because we are also part and parcel of the Supreme, we have partial blissfulness and eternality, and we are full of knowledge, according to our infinitesimal size.

The human beings are understood to be the most intelligent of all living creatures, but they are misusing their intelligence. How? They are misusing their intelligence by devoting it to the animal propensities. These animal propensities are eating, sleeping, mating and fearing. You can analyze the trend of modern civilization: everyone is busy with these four principles of animal life. They are sleeping and creating some cushions for comfortable sleep. They are creating palatable dishes for the eating propensity. They are exciting sex very nicely, for the mating necessity. And they are defending their country with so many atom bombs–that is the fear propensity.

But these symptoms you will find among the animals. They are also sleeping according to their own ways, and they are defending. They may not have the atom bomb, but they have some way of defending. You can kill your enemy, or he can kill you, but there is actually no defense. You cannot defend yourself; wherever you drop the bomb, it will hurt you, due to nuclear radiation. So this is not the solution of your problems. The solution of your problems is to get out of the conditioned state of life. That is called *yoga*—to link yourself to the Supreme.

There is a Supreme. This material creation is so nice—don't you think there is a friend behind it? The sky is so beautiful, the foodstuff is being produced, the moon is rising in due course, the sun is rising in due course, supplying heat for your health, supplying heat to the planetary systems. Everything is arranged very nicely; and yet the fools say there is no brain behind it, but it is all happening automatically.

The fact is that there is God, Kṛṣṇa, and we are all parts and parcels of Kṛṣṇa. We have been conditioned in some way or other in this material atmosphere. But now we have this human form of life, and so we have to get out of the entanglement. But getting out is not possible. You cannot get out of the entanglement of the material body unless you develop your Kṛṣṇa consciousness. Kṛṣṇa consciousness is not artificial—don't think that. This is the greatest necessity of the human being. Kṛṣṇa consciousness, God consciousness, is there within you. Don't you find, when there is a *kīrtana* performance, that the more innocent a person is, the sooner he begins? Immediately, the child begins to clap, begins to dance. This is within him; and it is very simple, this Kṛṣṇa consciousness.

So, unless you develop Kṛṣṇa consciousness, there is no rescue from the entanglement of conditioned life. This you have to understand. This is not some sentiment. No, it is a great science. You have to understand it nicely. Then the human form of life will be successful, and otherwise it is defeated. You may become a very great nation, but that is not the solution of the problem of life.

By the grace of Kṛṣṇa, I am able to serve you with my life's energy. I left the United States in 1967 in poor health; but life and death–everything–depends on Kṛṣṇa. I thought, "Let me go back to Vṛndāvana, because Vṛndāvana is a sanctified place where Kṛṣṇa consciousness is very strong." I thought that I might go there and die in Kṛṣṇa consciousness. Of course, if you are always in the atmosphere of Kṛṣṇa consciousness, then here also you can have Vṛndāvana. Vṛndāvana is not a particular place that is called Vṛndāvana. Kṛṣṇa says, "It is not that I live in the Kingdom of God, Vaikuṇṭha; nor is it that I live in the heart of the *yogī*." The *yogī* wants to find out where Kṛṣṇa is within the heart. But Kṛṣna says, "I am not in the abode in the spiritual sky, nor am I in the heart of the *yogī*." Then where are You? Kṛṣṇa says, "I stay where My pure devotees are chanting My glories." That is Vṛndāvana.

So, if that is Vṛndāvana, then I am there. There is no difference. Wherever there is electric light, there is electricity. It is naturally understood. Similarly, wherever there is Kṛṣṇa consciousness, it is Vṛndāvana. We can create Vṛndāvana by the mercy of Kṛṣṇa, if we chant Hare Kṛṣṇa. Perfect this Kṛṣṇa consciousness; try to understand the philosophy behind it. It is a science, not a bluff. We can speak from any angle of vision.

Kṛṣṇa consciousness is the great necessity of human society. Learn it and appreciate it, comprehend it and assimilate it—and teach it. It is very simple. If you offenselessly chant Hare Kṛṣṇa, everything will be revealed from within because Kṛṣṇa is sitting within you. If you are strong and have faith and conviction in Kṛṣṇa, as well as in the spiritual master, the transparent via medium to Kṛṣṇa, then Kṛṣṇa is there. The *Vedas* say that if you have implicit faith in God and implicit faith in your bona fide *guru*, who teaches you Kṛṣṇa consciousness, then the result will be that all the Vedic scriptures will be revealed authoritatively.

The process is spiritual; it does not require any material qualifications. The speculators who are not realized souls are covered in delusion and are simply wasting their time. Whatever they may do in their official class, they remain the same foolish rascals. But our Kṛṣṇa conscious students will feel a change in their lives, a change in happiness, and a change in youth, also. This is reality.

I shall request you, my dear young girls and boys, to take Kṛṣṇa consciousness very seriously, and you will be happy—your life will be perfected. It will be the sublime addition to your life. It is not a bluff. We have not come here to collect some money. Money is supplied by Kṛṣṇa. I am going back and forth to India—not only I, but my students as well. For a rich man there would be many expenditures; it would cost ten thousand dollars for such trips. But our business is Kṛṣṇa, and He will supply. I do not know where the money comes from, but Kṛṣṇa supplies. In Kṛṣṇa consciousness, you will be happy. You are the young generation; you are the flower of your country and society. Practice this most sublime system, Kṛṣṇa consciousness. Be happy and make others happy. This is the real mission of life.

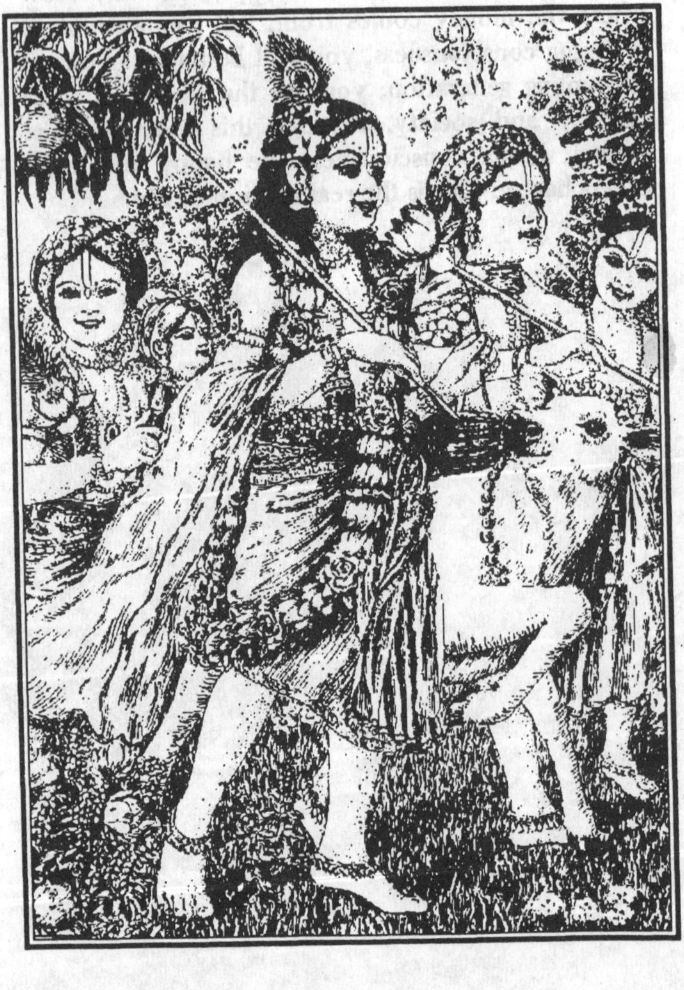

5
Our Real Life

The *Bhagavad-gītā* says that out of many thousands of human beings, one may try to make perfection of his life. Man is an animal, but he has one special prerogative, rational thought. What is that rational thought? Reasoning power, argument. Now, reasoning power is there in dogs and cats as well. Suppose a dog comes up to you; if you say, "Hut!" he'll understand. The dog will understand that you don't want him. So, he has some reasoning power. But what is the special reasoning power of the human being?

As far as the bodily necessities are concerned, the reasoning power is there even in the animal. If a cat wants to steal some milk from your kitchen, she has very nice reasoning power: she is always looking to see when the master is out and she can take. So, for the four propensities of animal life—eating, sleeping. mating and defending—there is reasoning power even in beasts. Then, what is the special reasoning power of the human being, by which he is called the rational animal?

The special reasoning power is to inquire, "Why am I suffering?" This is special reasoning. The animals are suffering, but they do not know how to remedy the suffering. But human beings are making scientific advancement and philosophical advancement, cultural advancement, religious advancement—progress in so many lines—because they want to be happy. "Where is the point of happiness?" This reasoning power is especially given to the human being. Therefore, in the *Gītā*, Kṛṣṇa says, "Out of so many men, one may know Me."

Generally, the people are just like animals. They simply do not know anything beyond the necessities of the body: how to eat, how to sleep, how to mate and how to defend. And the *Bhagavad-gītā* says, out of many thousands, someone may develop this reasoning power: "Why am I suffering?" He asks this question: "Why am I suffering?" We do not want to suffer, but suffering is forced upon us. We do not want too much cold, but too much cold and too much heat are forced upon us.

When there is some impetus to awaken this reasoning power, it is called *brahma-jijñāsā*. This is found in the *Vedānta-sūtra*. The first verse says that now, this human form of life is meant for asking the question of how to solve the problem of suffering.

So Kṛṣṇa says that this special prerogative of the human being is not awakened very easily, except by some good association. Just as we have this Kṛṣṇa conscious association. If we attain such association, where nice things are discussed, then that awakening of reason, that special prerogative of the human being, will come. As long as this question does not arise in one's mind, he should understand that whatever activities he is doing will lead to his defeat. He is simply leading an animal life. But, not when these questions arise: Why am I suffering? What am I? Am I meant for suffering? Am I meant for troubles?

I am undergoing troubles by nature's laws, and by the state's laws. So the question of freedom is how to become free from all these troubles. The *Vedānta-sūtra* also says that the soul, my actual self, is by nature joyful. Yet, I am suffering. Lord Kṛṣṇa further says that when these questions arise, gradually one comes to God. Those who have awakened to these questions are said to be on the path of perfection. And, when the question of God and our relationship with God comes, that is our final perfection of life.

Now, Kṛṣṇa says that out of many thousands of people, one may try to make perfection of this life; and out of many millions of such persons on the path of perfection, only one may understand Kṛṣṇa. So understanding Kṛṣṇa is not very easy. But it is also the easiest. It is not easy, but at the same time it is the easiest. It is the easiest if you follow the prescribed forms.

Lord Caitanya Mahāprabhu has introduced this chanting of Hare Kṛṣṇa. He has not exactly introduced it; it is in the scriptures. But He has especially propagated this formula. In this age this is the easiest method of self-realization. Simply chant Hare Kṛṣṇa. It can be done by everyone. In my classroom, I am perhaps the only Indian. My students are all Americans, and they are taking part in the chanting very nicely, chanting and dancing. That means that, in any country, in any place, this can be performed. Therefore it is the easiest. You may not understand the philosophy of the *Bhagavad-gītā*. That is also not very difficult; but still, if you think that you cannot understand, you can still chant very easily: Hare Kṛṣṇa, Hare Kṛṣṇa.

If we want to understand God, Kṛṣṇa, this is the beginning. The easiest beginning–simply chanting. Now, there are many students of my ISKCON institution. This institution is open a little over a year; but some of the students, by simply chanting, by the grace of Kṛṣṇa, have advanced in such a way that they can talk about the science of God, and they will very easily answer those human questions. So, this is the easiest method of transcendental meditation.

Kṛṣṇa says that out of many millions of people, one may understand Him. But, by chanting of this Hare Kṛṣṇa, as introduced by Lord Caitanya–chant ing and dancing–you can understand Kṛṣṇa within a very short time. Knowledge begins not from Kṛṣṇa, but from things which we are accustomed to see every day.

Land is gross. If you touch it, you can feel its hardness. But, as soon as the land becomes still finer, it is water, and the touch is soft. And then again, from water to fire, still finer. After fire or electricity the air is still finer; and after air, the sky, ether, is finer still. Beyond ether, the mind is still finer; and beyond the mind, intelligence is still finer. And, if you go beyond intelligence to understand the soul, it is finer still. From these elements people have discovered so many sciences. There are many scientists, for example, who are soil experts; they can say, by analyzing a particular type of earth, what kind of minerals are there. Somebody seeks out silver, somebody seeks out gold, somebody seeks out mica. This is knowledge of gross things—the earth. If you go to finer substances, then you study water, or liquid things, such as petrol and alcohol. Go still finer, and from water you will go to fire and electricity. If you study electricity, you have to study all sorts of books. And, from this finer fire, you will come to air. We have so much advancement in our airplanes; we are studying how they move, how they are made—now sputniks and jets—so many things are being discovered.

Next comes the study of the ethereal: electronics, ethereal transformations from one thing to another. Then, finer still, is the mind—psychology and psychiatry. But for intelligence, rationalism, there is only a little philosophical speculation. And what about the soul? Is there any science of the soul? The materialists have none. Material science has advanced to the study of the ether, or the mind and intelligence, but there is no advancement beyond that. Beyond intelligence, they do not know what exists. But here in the *Bhagavad-gītā* you can find this.

The *Bhagavad-gītā* begins at the point after intelligence. When Arjuna was perplexed at the outset, his intelligence was perplexed—whether to fight or not to fight. Kṛṣṇa begins the *Gītā* from the point where intelligence fails. How does knowledge of the soul begin? It is just like a child is playing. You can understand this child's body is now so small, but one day this child will be grown up, like you or me. But the same soul will continue. So, by intelligence, you can understand that although the body is changed, the soul is there. The same soul which was existing in the body of the child is still continuing in the body of the old man. Therefore the soul is permanent, and only the body has changed. This is a very easy thing to understand. And the last change of this body is death. As at every moment, every second, every day, every hour, the body is changing, so the last change is when one cannot act with the body, and so he has to take another one. Just as, when my cloth is too worn out or old, I cannot put it on; I have to take a new cloth. It is similar with the soul. When the body is too old or unworkable, I have to change to another body. This is called death.

This is the beginning of the *Bhagavad-gītā,* when the preliminary knowledge of the soul is there. And you will find that there are only a few who can understand the existence of the soul as permanent, and of the body as changeable. Therefore Bhagavān, Lord Kṛṣṇa, says that, out of many, many millions of people, one may understand it. But still, the knowledge is there. If you want to understand it, it is not difficult. You can understand it.

Now, we should inquire into the existence of the ego, the finest material substance. What is ego? I am pure soul, but with my intelligence and mind I am in contact with matter, and I have identified myself with matter. This is false ego. I am pure soul, but I am identifying falsely. For example, I am identifying with the land, thinking that I am Indian, or that I am American. This is called *ahaṅkara. Ahaṅkara* means the point where the pure soul touches matter. That junction is called *ahaṅkara. Ahaṅkara* is still finer than intelligence.

Kṛṣṇa says that these are the eight material elements: earth, water, fire, air, ether, mind, intelligence and false ego. False ego means false identification. Our nescient life has begun from this false identification—thinking that I am this matter, although I am seeing every day, at every moment, that I am not this matter. Soul is permanently existing, while matter is changing. This misconception, this illusion, is called *ahaṅkara*, false ego. And your liberation means when you are out of this false ego. What is that status? *Ahaṁ brahmāsmi.* I am *Brahman*, I am spirit. That is the beginning of liberation.

Of course, one may be suffering from disease, from fever, and the temperature may come down to normal, 98.6 degrees. So he is now normal, but that is not the cure. Suppose for two days he has a 98.6 degree temperature, but with a slight change of diet, a slight change of behavior, the temperature rises immediately to 100. Relapse. Similarly, simply purifying the mind, rejecting this false *ahaṅkara* identification—I am not this body, I am not this matter; I am soul—this is not liberation. It is only the beginning of liberation. If you stick to this point, and continue—just as you might continue your activities and keep your temperature at 98.6 degrees—then you are a healthy man.

For example, in the West now there is some propaganda for taking intoxication. The people want to forget the bodily existence. But how long will you forget? There will be a relapse. You can forget for one hour or two, by intoxication, and think that I am not this body. But unless you are actually on the platform of understanding yourself by knowledge, it is not possible to continue. Still, everyone is trying to think, "I am not this body." They have experience that they are suffering so much on account of bodily identification, and so, "If only I could forget my bodily identification!"

This is only a negative conception. When you actually realize yourself, simply understanding that you are *Brahman* will not do. You have to engage in the activities of *Brahman.* Otherwise you will fall down. Simply flying very high is no solution to the problem of going to the moon. Nowadays the fools are trying to go to the moon, but they simply go 240,000 miles up from the Earth, touch the moon, and return. They are very proud. There is so much talk of aeronautics: crowds and meetings and conferences. But what have they done? What are 240,000 miles in that vast sky? If you go 240 million miles, still you are limited. So this will not do. If you want to go high, you must have permanent shelter. If you can take rest there, then you cannot fall down. But if you have no rest, then you will have to fall down. The airplane goes high, seven miles, eight miles up from the earth, but it comes down immediately.

So, simply understanding *ahaṅkara* means no more than understanding the false identification. Simply understanding that I am not matter, I am soul, is not perfection. The impersonalist, the void philosopher, simply thinks of the negative, that I am not this matter, I am not this body. This will not stay. You have to not only realize that you are not matter, but you have to engage yourself in the spiritual world.

And that spiritual world means to be working in Kṛṣṇa consciousness. That spiritual world, that functioning of our real life, is Kṛṣṇa consciousness.

False ego I have already explained. It is neither matter nor spirit, but the junction—where the spirit soul comes into contact with matter and forgets himself. It is just as, in delirium, a man is diseased and his brain becomes puzzled, and gradually he forgets himself and becomes a madman. He is gradually forgetting. So there is the beginning of loss, and there is one point where he forgets. That beginning point is called *ahaṅkara,* or false ego

Chanting the *mahāmantra*—Hare Kṛṣṇa, Hare Kṛṣṇa, Kṛṣṇa Kṛṣṇa, Hare Hare/ Hare Rāma, Hare Rāma, Rāma Rāma, Hare Hare—is the process not merely of putting an end to this false conception of the self, but it goes beyond that, to the point where the pure spirit soul engages in his eternal, blissful, all-knowing activities in the loving service of God. This is the height of conscious development, the ultimate goal of all living entities now evolving through the cycles and species of material nature.

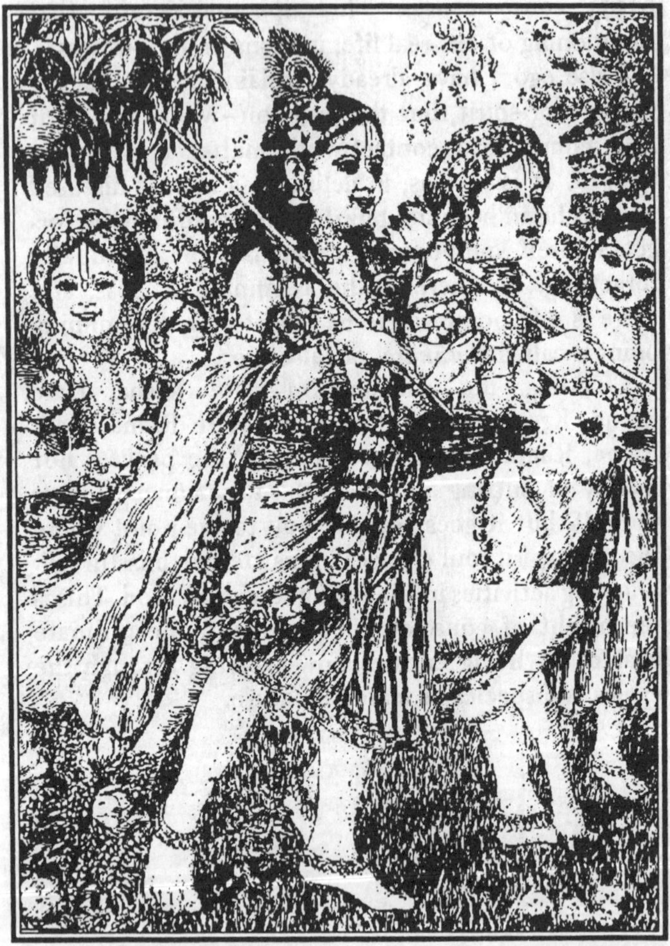

6
The Hare Kṛṣṇa Mantra

The transcendental vibration established by the chanting of HARE KṚṢṆA, HARE KṚṢṆA, KṚṢṆA KṚṢṆA, HARE HARE/ HARE RĀMA, HARE RĀMA, RĀMA RĀMA, HARE HARE is the sublime method for reviving our transcendental consciousness. As living spiritual souls, we are all originally Kṛṣṇa conscious entities, but due to our association with matter from time immemorial, our consciousness is now adulterated by the material atmosphere. The material atmosphere, in which we are now living, is called *māyā,* or illusion. *Māyā* means that which is not. And what is this illusion? The illusion is that we are all trying to be lords of material nature, while actually we are under the grip of her stringent laws. When a servant artificially tries to imitate the all-powerful master, it is called illusion. We are trying to exploit the resources of material nature, but actually we are becoming more and more entangled in her complexities. Therefore, although we are engaged in a hard struggle to conquer nature, we are ever more dependent on her. This illusory struggle against material nature can be stopped at once by revival of our eternal Kṛṣṇa consciousness.

Hare Kṛṣṇa, Hare Kṛṣṇa, Kṛṣṇa Kṛṣṇa, Hare Hare is the transcendental process for reviving this original pure consciousness. By chanting this transcendental vibration, we can cleanse away all misgivings within our hearts. The basic principle of all such misgivings is the false consciousness that I am the lord of all I survey.

Kṛṣṇa consciousness is not an artificial imposition on the mind. This consciousness is the original natural energy of the living entity. When we hear the transcendental vibration, this consciousness is revived. This simplest method of meditation is recommended for this age. By practical experience also, one can perceive that by chanting this *mahāmantra*, or the Great Chanting for Deliverance one can at once feel a transcendental ecstasy coming through from the spiritual stratum. In the material concept of life we are busy in the matter of sense gratification as if we were in the lower animal stage. A little elevated from this status of sense gratification, one is engaged in mental speculation for the purpose of getting out of the material clutches. A little elevated from this speculative status, when one is intelligent enough, one tries to find out the supreme cause of all causes—within and without. And when one is factually on the plane of spiritual understanding, surpassing the stages of sense, mind and intelligence, he is then on the transcendental plane. This chanting of the Hare Kṛṣṇa *mantra* is enacted from the spiritual platform, and thus this sound vibration surpasses all lower strata of consciousness—namely sensual, mental and intellectual. There is no need, therefore, to understand the language of the *mantra;* nor is there any need for mental speculation nor any intellectual adjustment for chanting this *mahāmantra.* It is automatic, from the spiritual platform, and as such, anyone can take part in vibrating this transcendental sound without any previous qualification. In a more advanced stage, of course, one is not expected to commit offenses on grounds of spiritual understanding.

In the beginning, there may not be the presence of all transcendental ecstasies, which are eight in number. These are: 1) Being stopped as though dumb, 2) perspiration, 3) standing up of hairs on the body, 4) dislocation of voice, 5) trembling, 6) fading of the body, 7) crying in ecstasy, and 8) trance. But there is no doubt that chanting for a while takes one immediately to the spiritual platform, and one shows the first symptom of this in the urge to dance along with the chanting of the *mantra*. We have seen this practically. Even a child can take part in the chanting and dancing. Of course, for one who is too entangled in material life, it takes a little more time to come to the standard point, but even such a materially engrossed man is raised to the spiritual platform very quickly. When it is chanted by a pure devotee of the Lord in love, it has the greatest efficacy on hearers, and as such this chanting should be heard from the lips of a pure devotee of the Lord, so that immediate effects can be achieved. As far as possible, chanting from the lips of nondevotees should be avoided. Milk touched by the lips of a serpent has poisonous effects.

The word *Harā* is the form of addressing the energy of the Lord, and the words *Kṛṣṇa* and *Rāma* are forms of addressing the Lord Himself. Both *Kṛṣṇa* and *Rāma* mean the supreme pleasure, and *Harā* is the supreme pleasure energy of the Lord, changed to

Hare (Hah-ray) in the vocative. The supreme pleasure energy of the Lord helps us to reach the Lord.

The material energy, called *māyā,* is also one of the multi-energies of the Lord. And we the living entities are also the energy, marginal energy, of the Lord. The living entities are described as superior to material energy. When the superior energy is in contact with the inferior energy, an incompatible situation arises; but when the superior marginal energy is in contact with the superior energy, called *Harā,* it is established in its happy, normal condition.

These three words, namely *Harā*, *Kṛṣṇa* and *Rāma,* are the transcendental seeds of the *mahāmantra.* The chanting is a spiritual call for the Lord and His energy, to give protection to the conditioned soul. This chanting is exactly like the genuine cry of a child for its mother's presence. Mother Harā helps the devotee achieve the Lord Father's grace, and the Lord reveals Himself to the devotee who chants this *mantra* sincerely.

No other means of spiritual realization is as effective in this age of quarrel and hyprocrisy as the *mahamantra:* Hare Kṛṣṇa, Hare Kṛṣṇa, Kṛṣṇa Kṛṣṇa, Hare Hare/ Hare Rāma, Hare Rāma, Rāma Rāma, Hare Hare.

7
How Bhakti-yoga Works

In the *Bhagavad-gītā* Kṛṣṇa tells His disciple, Arjuna, "I am disclosing a most confidential part of knowledge to you, because you are My dear friend." As is stated in the Fourth Chapter, the *Bhagavad-gītā* is spoken to Arjuna because of his one qualification: he was a devotee. The Lord says that the mystery of the *Bhagavad-gītā* is very confidential. Without being an unalloyed devotee you cannot know it. In India there are 645 different commentaries on the *Gītā.* One professor has proposed that Kṛṣṇa is a doctor and Arjuna is His patient and has made his commentary in that way. Similarly, there are commentators and people who have taken it that everyone is perfect, and that they can interpret scripture in their own way. As far as we are concerned, we agree to read the *Bhagavad-gītā* according to the instructions given in the *Gītā* itself. This has to be taken through the *paramparā,* the system of disciplic succession. It is being taught by the Supreme Person because "you are My dear friend. I desire that you may become prosperous and happy. Therefore I speak to you." Kṛṣṇa wants everyone to be happy and peaceful and prosperous, but they do not want it. Sunshine is open to everyone, but if someone wishes to remain in darkness, what can the sunshine do for him? So the *Gītā* is open to everyone. There are different species of life, and lower and higher grades of understanding exist—that is a fact.

But Kṛṣṇa says that this knowledge is for anyone. If one has lower birth or whatever, it doesn't matter. The *Bhagavad-gītā* offers transcendental subject matter everyone can understand provided he goes along with the principle as stated in the Fourth Chapter. That is, that the *Gītā* is coming down in disciplic succession: "I first of all instructed this *yoga* system to the sun-god Vivasvān, who taught it to Manu, who taught it to Ikṣvāku." From Kṛṣṇa the disciplic succession is coming down, but "in course of time the disciplic succession was broken." Arjuna is therefore made the new disciple. In the Second Chapter, Arjuna surrenders: "So far we have been talking as friends, but now I accept You as my spiritual master." Anyone following the principle in this line accepts the *guru* as Kṛṣṇa, and the student must represent Arjuna. Kṛṣṇa is speaking as the spiritual master of Arjuna, and Arjuna says, "Whatever You are saying I accept." Read it like that–not: "I like this, so I accept it; this I don't like, and so I reject it." Such reading is useless nonsense.

The teacher must be a representative of Kṛṣṇa, a devotee, and the student must be like Arjuna. Then this Kṛṣṇa consciousness study is perfect. Otherwise it is a waste of time. In the *Śrīmad-Bhāgavatam* it is stated: "If anyone wants to understand the science of Kṛṣṇa, he should associate with pure devotees. When discussions take place among pure devotees, the potency of spiritual language is revealed." Scholarly discussion of the *Gītā* is futile. In the *Upaniṣads* it is stated: "To one who has firm faith in God, and similar faith in God's representative, all the import of

Vedic language will be revealed." We must have the qualification of being a devotee. Become dear to God. My spiritual master used to say, "Don't try to see God. Act in such a way that God will see you." We have to qualify ourselves. By your qualification God Himself will come and see you.

If one can perceive God, he is transcendental to all material demands. We are always dissatisfied in the material world in circumstances that won't continue; happiness is temporary, and temporary plight also will not exist for much time. Cold, heat, duality—it is all coming and going. To get to the absolute stage is the process of Kṛṣṇa consciousness. Kṛṣṇa is seated in everyone's heart, and as you become purified He will show you the path. And in the end you will quit this body, and you will go to the spiritual sky.

"No one knows Me," Kṛṣṇa says, "My influence, My power and My extent. Even the *maharṣis* [the great thinkers] don't know. I am the origin of all demigods and the origin of all *ṛṣis."* There are so many forefathers we don't know of, and there are Brahmā and the demigods—what do we know? We can't reach to the platform where we can grasp God. We gather knowledge by limited senses, and Kṛṣṇa can't be reached by the mind, the center of the senses. Imperfect senses can't grasp perfect knowledge. Mind and sense manipulation can't reach Him. If you engage the senses in the service of the Lord, however, then He will reveal Himself through your senses.

People may say, "What is the use of understanding God? What is the use? Let Him stay in His place, let me stay in my place." But in the *śāstras*, the scriptures, it is stated that pious activities will raise us to beauty, knowledge and good birth; and that by impious (sinful) activities, we suffer. Suffering is always there, pious or impious, but a distinction is made. He who knows God, however, becomes freed from all possible sinful reactions, which no amount of piety can accomplish. If we reject God we can never be happy.

Not even considering human society, if you take the demigods who are more advanced and intelligent, they also don't know Kṛṣṇa. The seven great sages whose planet is near the North Star also do not know. Kṛṣṇa says: "I am the original, the source of all these demigods." He is the father of everything, not only the origin of demigods, but of the sages—and the universe. The *Śrīmad-Bhāgavatam* describes how the universal form took place, and everything is emanating from Him. Also Kṛṣṇa is the origin of *Paramātmā*, the Supersoul; and the impersonal *brahmajyoti*, the shining effulgence, is in Him. Of everything, of every conception, "I am the source." The Absolute Truth may be realized in three phases, but is one nondual truth. *Brahman* (the glowing effulgence), localized Supersoul, and *Bhāgavan*—the Supreme Person—are three features or aspects of God.

If no one knows the Supreme Personality of Godhead, how can He be known? He can be known when the Supreme Lord comes before you and reveals Himself to you. Then you can know. Our senses are imperfect, and they cannot realize the Supreme Truth. When you adopt a submissive attitude and chant, realization begins from the tongue. To eat and to vibrate sound is the business of the tongue. If you can control your tongue for *prasādam*, spiritual food, and make the sound vibration of the holy name, then by surrender of the tongue you can control all the other senses. If you cannot control your tongue, you cannot control your senses. Taste *prasādam* and become spiritually advanced. You can have this process at your home: offer vegetarian foods to Kṛṣṇa, chant the Hare Kṛṣṇa *mantra* and offer obeisances:

namo brahmaṇya-devāya
go-brāhmaṇa-hitāya ca
jagat-hitāya kṛṣṇāya
govindāya namo namaḥ

Everyone can offer, and then take the food with friends. And chant before the picture of Kṛṣṇa, and lead a pure life. Just see the result—the whole world will become Vaikuṇṭha, where there is no anxiety. All is anxious with us because we have accepted this material life. Just the opposite is so in the spiritual world. No one, however, knows how to get out of the material concept. Taking an intoxicant doesn't help; the same anxieties are there when you are finished being drunk. If you want to be free and want life eternal with bliss and knowledge, take to Kṛṣṇa. No one can know God, but there is this way: the process of Kṛṣṇa consciousness.

In the *Śrīmad-Bhāgavatam* it is stated that no one can conquer Him or approach Him, but He becomes conquered. How? Let people remain in their own positions, but let them give up nonsense speculation through volumes of books. Thousands of books are printed and read, and after six months thrown away. This way and that—how can you know the Supreme by speculation on the information supplied by your blunt senses? Give up research—throw it away—just become submissive; acknowledge that you are limited and subordinate to material nature and to God. No one can be equal to or greater than God So be submissive. Try to hear about the glories of the Supreme Lord from authorized sources. Such authority is handed over by disciplic succession. If we can understand by the same authority as Arjuna, that is real authority. God is always ready to reveal; you just become Kṛṣṇa conscious. Follow the path traversed by the great *ācāryas,* the devoted teachers, and then everything will be known. Although He is unconquerable and unknowable, He can be known in your home.

If you take to this process and follow the principles, what will be the result? As soon as you understand, you will know that the Supreme Lord is the cause of all causes, but that He is not caused by any other cause. And He is the master of all planets. This is not accepting blindly. God has given you the power of reason, the power of arguing—but don't argue falsely. If you want to know the transcendental science you must surrender. Surrender to authority and know Him by signs. Don't surrender to a fool or a rascal. Find one who is coming in disciplic succession, one who is fully convinced about the Supreme Absolute

Truth. If you find such a person, surrender and try to please him, serve him and question him. Surrender unto Him is surrender to God. Question to learn, not to waste time.

The process is there, but if we waste time by intoxication we will never see Him, the unconquerable Lord. Follow the principles and slowly but surely, without doubt, you will know. "Yes, I'm making progress," you'll say. And it is very easy, and you can execute it and be in a happy mood. Study, take part with music, eat *prasādam*. And no one can cheat you by this process. But if you want to be cheated—go to the cheaters.

Try to understand it from the authoritative source and apply it in your life. Amongst the dying mortals, you will become the most intelligent because you are freed from sinful actions. If you act only for Kṛṣṇa, then you are freed from all reactions. You will have no anxiety over what is auspicious or inauspicious because you will be in touch with the most auspicious. This is the process. Ultimately, we can get in touch with Kṛṣṇa. Life will be successful. Anyone can adopt it, because it is very simple.

Here is a nice formula presented by Kṛṣṇa Himself: one should understand the position of Kṛṣṇa. He is unborn and without any cause. We have experience, all of us, that we are born, and we have a cause; our father is our cause. If someone poses himself as God, he has to prove that he is unborn and uncaused. Our practical experience is that we are born. Kṛṣṇa is not born. We have to understand this. Understanding this is to be firmly convinced He is the cause, but is not caused; and since He is not caused He is the proprietor of all manifestation. One who understands this simple philosophy is not illusioned.

We are generally illusioned. We are claiming ownership of the land. But before my birth the land was here, and after my death it will still be here. How long will I go on claiming, in body after body, "This is my land! This is my land!"? Is it not nonsense? One has to be out of illusion. We should know that whatever we are doing in the material concept of life is illusion. We have to understand whether we are illusioned or not. And all conditioned souls are illusioned. He who learns to be disillusioned gets free of all encumbrances. If we want freedom from all bonds, then we have to understand God. There is no neglecting this; it is our prime duty.

Out of millions of entities, one may be enlightened. Generally we are all born fools. As soon as I take birth I am nurtured by parents and educated to falsely claim a land as my own. National education means to make you more foolish. Am I not foolish? I am changing my body like a dress life after life. You have so many minds, so many dresses—why do you claim this one? Why don't you understand: "This dress is nice, but next moment I may be in another." You are in the grip of nature. You cannot say what dress you will have: "Nature, make me American." No; material nature controls. If you live like a dog—here, take a dog's dress. If you live a godly life—here, take God.

Out of many fools someone tries to understand what I actually am. Dog? American? Russian? This real inquiry goes on. If you inquire, you have to ask someone, not just yourself. When crossing the street in a place you don't know, you have to ask the policeman or some gentleman. For "what I am" you have to go to an authority also. What is a spiritual master? He is a person conversant with the science of Kṛṣṇa. Ordinarily nobody inquires; but if a man does, he can make progress and come to this understanding: Kṛṣṇa is the cause of all causes.

Four kinds of people, followers of scripture and higher authority, inquire about Kṛṣṇa. Those addicted to sinful activities can't inquire. They go on in intoxication. The righteous, pious man inquires and goes to God. Facility is given to people in this process by the authority—to make people happy, not to exploit people. The purpose of ISKCON is, in this way, to understand the science of God. You want happiness. Here it is. You are distressed by sinful reactions. But if there is no sinful reaction there is no suffering. One who knows Kṛṣṇa without doubt is relieved of all reactions. Kṛṣṇa says, "Come to Me, and I will give you freedom from all reactions." Don't disbelieve it. He can give you shelter; He has all power. If I give you such a promise, because I have no such power I may break the promise.

If you associate yourself with Kṛṣṇa consciousness your dormant relationship with Kṛṣṇa will be evoked. You have a relationship with Him. There is no question of disbelieving; it is simply foolishness. The dormant relationship is there. You want to serve Kṛṣṇa, but simply by the spell of illusion we think we have no connection with Kṛṣṇa. We go on doing all "independent" nonsense, and we are always anxious. When we associate with these dormant feelings for Krsna, however, we will become engaged in Kṛṣṇa consciousness.

"God is unborn" indicates that He is different from the material world. We have no such experience of the unborn. This city was born–history is filled with dates. Spiritual nature, however, is unborn, and at once we can see the difference. The material nature is born. You have to understand; if Kṛṣṇa is unborn then He is spiritual, not like one of us. Kṛṣṇa is not some "extraordinary person who was also born." He is not born. So how can I decide He is an ordinary man? "Those who are fools and rascals think of Me as an ordinary man," Kṛṣṇa says in the *Gītā.* He is different from everything in this world. He is *anādi,* without cause.

Kṛṣṇa may be spiritual, but there are other spiritual bodies. We have spiritual bodies like Kṛṣṇa's, but they are born. They are not exactly born; it is like the sparks of the fire. The sparks are not born from the fire; they are actually there. We are also not born; we are sparks that come out of the original form. Even if we are not born, the spark comes out of Kṛṣṇa, so we are different; the sparks of the fire are fire, but they are not the original fire. As for quality, we are the same as Kṛṣṇa. It is like the difference between father and son. Father and son are different and nondifferent at the same time. The son is an expansion of the father, but he cannot claim that he is the father; that would be nonsense.

Because Kṛṣṇa is declaring Himself supreme proprietor, He is therefore different from anything. If I am the proprietor of New York State, I am still not New York State. In every step there is dualtiy. No one can say we are completely one with God.

When you can understand Kṛṣṇa's and your own position in a nice analytical way, then at once you become free from sinful reactions. This process will help you. Chant Hare Kṛṣṇa and cleanse your mind, and you will receive the message. One has to be qualified. If you chant and hear, for no payment, you will approach God. All things will become clear and illuminated.

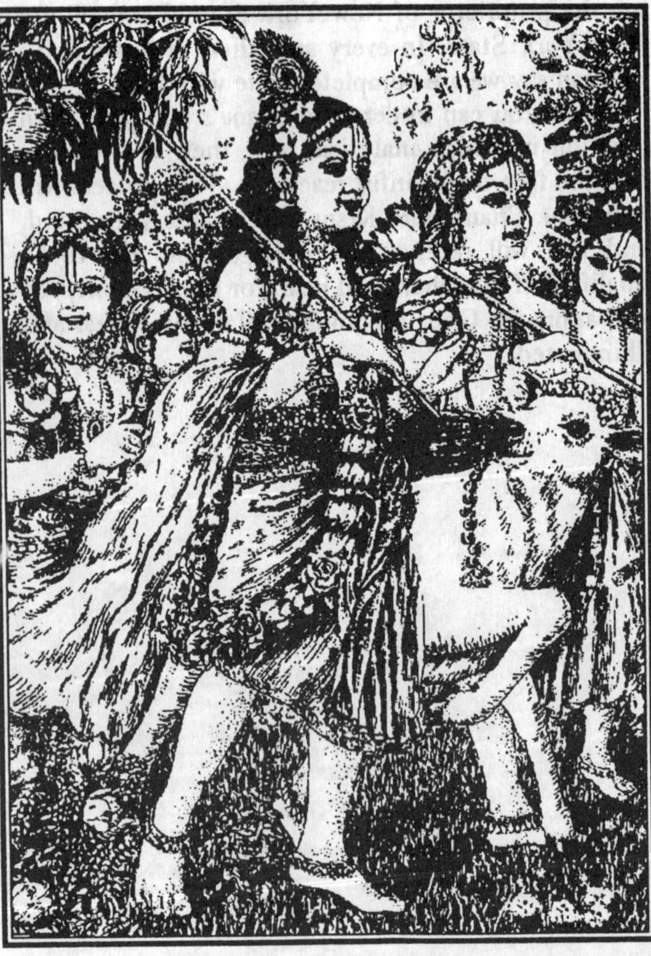

8
Sources of Absolute Knowledge

We require to hear about the method of relishing the *Śrīmad-Bhāgavatam,* the most elevated text on the science of God consciousness, the matured and ripened fruit of the tree of Vedic wisdom. The Sanskrit word *rasa* means juice, just like the juice of an orange or a mango. And the author of the *Śrīmad-Bhāgavatam* requests that you kindly try to taste the *rasa*, or juice, of the fruit of the *Bhāgavatam.* Why? Why shall I taste the juice of the fruit of the *Bhāgavatam*? Because it is the ripened fruit of the Vedic desire tree. As a desire tree, whatever you want you can have from the *Vedas. Veda* means knowledge; it is so complete that whether you want to enjoy in this material world or you want to enjoy spiritual life, both kinds of knowledge are there. If you follow the Vedic principles, then you will be happy. This is like the codes of the state. If the citizens obey, then they will be happy, there will be no criminal trespassing, and they will enjoy life. The state does not come to you for nothing just to trouble you, but if you live according to the state law there is no question of unhappiness.

Similarly, this conditioned soul, the living entity, has come here to this material world for enjoyment and for material happiness. And the *Vedas* are the guidance: all right, enjoy—but you enjoy according to these principles. That is called *Veda.* Therefore, everything is there. Just as we sometimes perform a marriage ceremony in the temple. What is this marriage ceremony? It is the combination of man and woman, boy and girl. They are already there, they are living like friends—what is the use of this marriage ceremony? It is Vedic: the *Vedas* account for living together, sex life, but under some special regulations so that you may be happy. The ultimate end is to become happy. If you follow the Vedic rules and restrictions, that will not mean that you will be kept from eating or not allowed to sleep, not allowed to defend or to have sex life. It is not like that. Your bodily necessities are the same as those of the animals; the animals also eat, they also sleep, they also mate and also defend. So we require these things also. But the *Vedas* prescribe some regulations: you act in this way, so that you will not be unhappy. If you follow the regulation, ultimately the result will be that you will be free from the material entanglement.

This material life is not meant for the spirit soul. It is simply a misunderstanding that you want to enjoy this material life. But Kṛṣṇa, the Supreme Lord, gives us specific orders so that we can enjoy, in such a way that, at the end, we will understand that this is not our proper life—our proper life is spiritual. This human form of life is perfected as soon as we come to the understanding of spiritual existence—that I am *Brahman.* Otherwise, if I do not take care of my spiritual life, then the result is that I must live as the cats and dogs do. There is every possibility that my next life will be an animal life. And if, by chance or by a freak of nature, I get into animal life, then millions and millions of years will be required before again coming to this human form of life. So the human form of life is meant for self-realization, and the *Vedas* are the direction.

Now in the *Bhagavad-gītā* you will find that Kṛṣṇa says that to study or to follow the rules and regulations of the *Vedas* actually means to come to the understanding of Kṛṣṇa consciousness. That is stated in the *Śrīmad-Bhāgavatam* also. So the *Vedas* give you the chance to gradually come to the point of understanding Kṛṣṇa, after many, many births. But the *Bhāgavatam* is called the essence of life, the ripened fruit of the *Vedas*, because the *Bhāgavatam* gives you directly what is needed in your life.

The *Vedas* are divided into four: *Sāma, Ṛk, Atharva* and *Yajus*. Then these are explained by the *Purāṇas*, of which there are eighteen. Then these are still further explained by the *Upaniṣads*, of which there are 108. The *Upaniṣads* are summarized in the *Vedānta-sūtra*, and the *Vedānta-sūtra* is still again explained by the *Śrīmad-Bhāgavatam*, by the same author. This is the process. So the *Bhāgavatam* is the essence of all Vedic knowledge.

Naimiṣāraṇya is a very famous and sacred forest in northern India, where all the *ṛṣis*, the sages, generally go to aid their spiritual advancement of life. This *Śrīmad-Bhāgavatam* was first discussed in this age in that forest. When it was discussed, the great saint Sūta Gosvāmī was asked by his audience: Now that Kṛṣṇa has gone back to His abode, with whom is transcendental knowledge now resting? This question was raised. The *Bhagavad-gītā* was spoken by Kṛṣṇa

Himself, and it contains all descriptions of *jñāna-yoga, karma-yoga, dhyāna-yoga* and *bhakti-yoga.* Now this inquiry was made: Where can you get spiritual knowledge, now that Kṛṣṇa is gone? The answer was that Kṛṣṇa, having departed, has left us the *Śrīmad-Bhāgavatam.* It is the representation, the sound representation, of Kṛṣṇa. The *Bhāgavatam* is not different from Kṛṣṇa, as the *Gītā* is not different from Kṛṣṇa. They are absolute. Kṛṣṇa and Kṛṣṇa's sound vibration are not different. Kṛṣṇa and Kṛṣṇa's name are also not different. And Kṛṣṇa and Kṛṣṇa's form, again, are not different. This is absolute. It requires realization.

This *Bhagavad-gītā* and *Śrīmad-Bhāgavatam* are sound incarnations of Kṛṣṇa. The *Śrīmad-Bhāgavatam* is also the literary incarnation of Kṛṣṇa, and it is the fruit of Vedic knowledge. You may have experience that there is a bird which is called a parrot. The parrot's body is green, and his beak is red. The specific qualification of the parrot is that whatever you say he can imitate. That parrot bird is touching the ripened fruit, and, naturally, if the fruit is ripened on the tree, it becomes very tasteful. Again, if the fruit is tasted by the parrot, it becomes still more tasteful. That is nature's way. So, here, it is said that this *Śrīmad-Bhāgavatam* is just like the ripened fruit of Vedic knowledge, and at the same time it is touched by Śukadeva Gosvāmī, Sūta's spiritual master. *Śuka* means parrot in Sanskrit.

This *Śrīmad-Bhāgavatam* was first explained by Śukadeva Gosvāmī, though the author is his father, Vyāsa. Śukadeva was only sixteen years old when he was taught the *Bhāgavatam*, and he was illumined. He was already liberated in the impersonal concept of the Absolute, but after hearing the *Bhāgavatam* from his father, he became attracted by the pastimes of Kṛṣṇa, and he became a preacher of the *Bhāgavatam*. First he explained it before Mahārāja Parīkṣit, the great king. A short history of Mahārāja Parīkṣit is that he was a very pious king, but unfortunately by some of his acts he was cursed by a *brāhmaṇa* boy to die within seven days. In those days if a *brāhmaṇa* should curse someone it would come true. They had the power to curse or give benediction.

So Parīkṣit understood that within a week he would have to die, and he prepared himself. He gave up his kingdom, entrusting it to his son, Mahārāja Janamejaya, and he detached himself from the family and sat down on the banks of the Ganges near Delhi. It was not exactly the Ganges; it was actually the Yamunā. There, because he was a great emperor, many learned sages came.

Parīkṣit now inquired from all the great sages present there: "What is my duty? I am going to die within seven days; now what is my duty? You are all learned sages; please just prescribe for me." So someone said to practice *yoga*, some said to practice *jñāna*, the cultivation of knowledge; there were different opinions. But at that time Śukadeva Gosvāmī entered the forest, and although Śukadeva was only sixteen, he was so learned and reputed that all the old sages, including his father, Vyāsadeva, stood up to show him respect. He was so learned. So when he appeared, it was agreed. "Here is Śukadeva Gosvāmī. Let him decide what to do. We appoint him as our representative."

Śukadeva Gosvāmī was thus authorized to speak, and he was asked, "What is my duty? I am very fortunate that you have come in this momentous hour. Kindly tell me what is my duty."

Śukadeva Gosvāmī said, "All right, I shall explain to you the *Śrīmad-Bhāgavatam.*" Then everyone present agreed.

As the *Bhāgavatam* was first spoken by Śukadeva Gosvāmī, it is therefore mentioned that as the parrot touches ripened fruit and it becomes even sweeter, so this *Śrīmad-Bhāgavatam,* because it was touched first by Śukadeva Gosvāmī, has become still more tasteful.

The idea is that any Vedic literature, especially the *Bhāgavatam* or the *Gītā,* should be learned as spoken by a realized soul. Especially this literature, which is called *Vaiṣṇava* literature. should not be heard from a person who is not a devotee. This point I have several times stressed. Those who are nondevotees, those who are mental speculationists, those who are fruitive workers, those who are meditators or mystic *yogīs,* cannot explain the science of God. This is especially mentioned also by Sanātana Gosvāmī, another great saint; those who are not in devotional service, nongodly, those who have no faith in God—such persons should not be allowed to speak on the *Bhagavad-gītā* and *Śrīmad-Bhāgavatam,* or any literature which is in relationship with the Supreme Lord. So it is not that anybody can speak the *Bhāgavatam* or the *Gītā* and we will have to hear it. No. Sanātana Gosvāmī especially prohibits us: we should not hear of the Supreme Lord from one who is not purified.

One may ask, "How can you taint the words of Kṛṣṇa, which are naturally transcendentally pure? What is the harm if we hear from the nondevotee?" This question may be raised. The example given here is that milk is very nice and nutritious, but as soon as it is touched by a serpent it becomes poison immediately. The serpent is very envious. He bites and puts to death immediately, unnecessarily, and therefore is considered the cruelest animal amongst the living entites. In the *sāstra* nonviolence is recommended, as in every scripture, but the serpent and the scorpion are allowed to be killed. You cannot say that milk is so nutritious, and we can drink—what is the harm if it is touched by serpents? No—the result will be death. One should not hear at least the *Bhagavad-gītā* and the *Śrīmad-Bhāgavatam* from those who are not devotees of the Lord, who have no realization of God and who are envious of Him. Their touch renders it poison. The words of the Lord are always sublime, but as soon as they are touched by the serpent-like nondevotee, one should be very careful about hearing.

In the *Bhāgavatam,* it is indicated that as soon as Śukadeva touched it, it became delicious. This is the distinction. Basically it is the ripened fruit of Vedic knowledge, but at the same time it has been touched by Śukadeva Gosvāmī.

The Lord is the supreme object of *yoga* and the reservoir of all transcendental pleasure; He reveals

Himself only to His devotees and by the mercy of His devotees all can relish His intimate association.

9
The Real Peace Formula

Every living entity is searching after peace. That is the struggle for existence. Everyone, from the aquatics to the highest form of human being—from the ant up to Brahmā, the first creature of this universe—is searching for peace. That is the main objective. Lord Caitanya said that a person who is in full Kṛṣṇa consciousness is the only peaceful man because he has no demands. That is the special qualification of a person who is in Kṛṣṇa consciousness. He is *akāmaḥ*. *Akāmaḥ* refers to those who have no desire, who are self-sufficient, who have nothing to ask and who are fully peaceful. Who are they? They are the devotees who are situated in Kṛṣṇa consciousness.

All others fall into three classes. One class is *bhukti*, those who are hankering after material happiness and enjoyment. These people want to eat, drink, be merry and enjoy. There are different modes of enjoyment according to the body. People are searching after sense enjoyment on this planet, on other planets, here, there and everywhere. Their main object is to gratify the senses. That is called *bhukti*. The next class is those people who are fatigued or frustrated in sense gratification and therefore want liberation from this material entanglement. And then there are those who, in search of knowledge, speculate about what the Absolute Truth is. Thus there are some who want sense enjoyment, and others, the salvationists, who are seeking liberation.

The salvationists also have some desire, the desire to be free from this material entanglement. Then there are those who are *yogīs;* they are searching after mystic perfection. There are eight kinds of mystic perfection which grant the ability to become the smallest, to become the heaviest, or to get whatever one desires. Ordinary persons who are after sense gratification and those who are salvationists or who are after mystic perfection all have some demand. But what about the devotees? They have no demands. Because they simply want to serve Kṛṣṇa, they are waiting for the order of Kṛṣṇa, and that is their satisfaction. If Kṛṣṇa wants the devotees to go to hell, they are prepared to go to hell. And if Kṛṣṇa says, "You come to Me," they are prepared to go. They have no demands. This is the perfectional stage.

There is a very nice verse in which a devotee prays: "I shall simply be conscious of You, my dear Lord, Kṛṣṇa conscious, free from all mental demands." Actually, because we are in material bondage, we have many demands. Some people want sense gratification, those who are a little more elevated want mental satisfaction, and those who are still more refined want to show some magic jugglery of power in this world. They are all in material bondage in different capacities. Therefore, a person who is Kṛṣṇa conscious prays to the Lord: "My dear Lord, when shall I be fully absorbed in Your thoughts or Your service?" "Your thoughts" are not simply abstract, concocted speculation; it is a practical mode of thought. "I shall become peaceful." All mental concoction—I want this, I want that—will be completely eradicated.

We are hovering over the mental plane. We have given power of attorney to the mind, and the mind is driving us—"Come here, go there." One has to stop such nonsense. "I shall simply be Your eternal servitor. And I shall be very cheerful, for I have my master." All others who are not in Kṛṣṇa consciousness are guideless. They are their own guides. The person who is Kṛṣṇa conscious has the supreme guide; therefore, he has no fear. For example, as long as a child is under the care of his parents he has no fear. But as soon as he becomes free, he finds many impediments. This is a crude example, but similarly, when one becomes completely free from all mental concoction and engages one hundred percent in Kṛṣṇa consciousness twenty-four hours a day, he will be peaceful at once. That is peace.

Therefore, Caitanya Mahāprabhu says that those who are Kṛṣṇa conscious, because they have no demands, are actually peaceful. Those who are after sense enjoyment, salvation and yogic mystic perfection are always full of anxiety. As long as one is full of anxiety, one should know that he is still under the grip of material nature. And as soon as one is free from all anxiety, one should know that he is liberated. This fearful anxiety exists because we do not know Kṛṣṇa, the Supreme Lord, the supreme controller. Instead, we have other conceptions, and therefore we are always anxious.

There are many examples, such as Prahlāda Mahārāja. He was only five years old, a pet child, but because he was a devotee of the Lord, his father became his enemy. This is the way of the world. As soon as one becomes a devotee of the Lord he finds so many obstacles. But those obstacles will not hinder one or be impediments on the path. We should always be personally prepared to become Kṛṣṇa conscious. Otherwise, there is only the kingdom of *māyā*, illusion. *Māyā* will try to defeat us as soon as she sees, "Oh, here is a living soul going out of my grip." As soon as one becomes Kṛṣṇa conscious and fully surrenders unto the Supreme Lord, he has nothing more to fear from this illusion. The Kṛṣṇa conscious person is the perfectly peaceful person.

Everyone wants peace in the world. The peace marchers do not know how to obtain peace, but they want peace. I read a speech of the Archbishop of Canterbury in which he said, "You want the kingdom of God without God." This is our defect. If you want peace at all, then accept that peace means to understand God. That is stated in the *Bhagavad-gītā.* Unless you are in touch with the Supreme Lord, Kṛṣṇa, you cannot have peace. Therefore, we have a different peace formula. The real peace formula is that one must know that God is the proprietor of all this universe, including the United States of America. He is the proprietor of Russia, He is the proprietor of China, He is the proprietor of India, of everything. But because we claim that we are the proprietors, there is fighting, there is discord, there is disagreement, and how can there be peace?

First of all, one has to accept that God is the proprietor of everything. We are simply guests for fifty or a hundred years. We come and go, and while one is here, he is absorbed in this thought: "This is my land. This is my family. This is my body. This is my property." And when there is an order from the Supreme for one to leave his home, his property, his body, his family, his money and his bank balance and it is all gone, one has to take another place. We are under the grip of material nature, and she is offering different kinds of bodies: "Now, my dear sir, you accept this body." We accept an American body, an Indian body, a Chinese body, a cat's body or a dog's body. I am not the proprietor even of this body, yet I say that I am this body. Actually, this is ignorance. And how can one have peace? Peace can be had when one understands that God is the proprietor of everything. One's friends, one's mother, one's mother's father and the President are all guests of time. When this knowledge is accepted, then there will be peace.

We are searching for a friend to give us peace and tranquility. That friend is Kṛṣṇa, God. Just make friendship with Him; you'll find everyone to be your friend. Because God is situated in everyone's heart, if you make friendship with God, He will dictate from within so that you will also be treated in a friendly way. If you make friendship with the police commissioner, you receive some advantage. If you make friendship with President Nixon, everyone will be your friend because everyone is under the President. If you want something from any officer, simply call President Nixon, and he will say, "All right, look after this man." Everything is taken care of. Just try to have friendship with God, and everyone will be your friend. If all people understand this very nice fact, that God is everyone's friend and that He is the supreme proprietor, they will become peaceful. That is explained also by Lord Caitanya.

In *Bhagavad-gītā, Śrīmad-Bhāgavatam, Caitanya-caritāmṛta,* or any Vedic literature or any other literature in any other religion, the same fact is presented: God is the proprietor. God is the only friend. If you understand this, then you'll have peace. This is the peace formula. As soon as you encroach on God's property, calling it your own, material nature, the police action, will be there: "You are not the proprietor." You can simply have what is allotted to you by God.

Your business is to elevate yourself to perfect Kṛṣṇa consciousness and nothing more. If you deviate from this law, if you don't accept this principle, if you want to enjoy more, then you have to suffer more. There is no question of forgetting. Therefore, Lord Caitanya says, "One who is Kṛṣṇa conscious has no demands. Thus he is at peace."

Those in Kṛṣṇa consciousness do not know anything more than Kṛṣṇa. Actually only those who are Kṛṣṇa conscious are peaceful, unafraid of anything. They are neither in heaven nor in hell nor anywhere but with Kṛṣṇa, so for them everything is Vaikuṇṭha, without fear. Similarly, Lord Kṛṣṇa as Paramātmā, Supersoul, lives everywhere. He lives in the heart of a hog also. The hog eats stool, but that does not mean that because the Supreme Lord is in the heart of the hog, He is also subjected to such punishment. The Lord and His devotees are always transcendental to the modes of material nature. Persons who are completely Kṛṣṇa conscious are very rare and very peaceful. Out of millions and millions of people, it is very difficult to find one who is actually Kṛṣṇa conscious; this position of Kṛṣṇa consciousness is so rare. But Kṛṣṇa Himself, as Lord Caitanya, seeing the pitiable condition of the present day, is directly giving free love of Godhead.

Yet because love of God is being given freely and so easily, people do not care for it. My spiritual master used to say that if you take a *langera* mango, which is a first-class, topmost quality mango in India, very costly, very sweet and very tasteful, and go from door to door and try to distribute it freely, people will doubt: "Why has this man brought this *langera* mango? Why is he trying to distribute it freely? There must be some motive behind it." Similarly, Lord Caitanya distributed this Kṛṣṇa consciousness *langera* mango very cheaply, but people are so foolish that they think, "Oh, they are simply chanting Hare Kṛṣṇa; what is there to it? This is meant for the foolish, who cannot speculate and do not have any higher standard of knowledge." But that is not so. It is said: "Out of millions and millions of people, only a few are interested in Kṛṣṇa consciousness." Do not neglect this information; it is very rare, and if you practice Kṛṣṇa consciousness, your life will be successful. Your mission in human life will be fulfilled. This seed of Kṛṣṇa consciousness is very rare and very valuable. Lord Caitanya said that innumerable living entities are wandering and transmigrating in the 8,400,000 species of life, one after another. Out of so many, one may come who is fortunate, who has spiritual fortune.

Sometimes devotees of the Lord go from door to door. Their policy is to go as beggars. So in India, beggars, especially *sannyāsīs,* are very much respected. If a *sannyāsī* comes to a house to beg, he is very well received: "Swamījī, what can I do for you?" The devotee beggar won't ask for anything, but whatever one can give, even one *capati,* makes one spiritually rich. That man who offers a *capati* to a pure devotee who comes to his door is made spiritually rich. When one is advanced in spiritual wealth, he offers a good reception to devotees as far as possible. According to the Vedic system, even if your enemy comes to your house, you have to receive him in such a way that you will forget that he is your enemy. That is the general system for receiving a pure devotee who has sacrificed everything for the Lord.

These are instructions for householders. The householder should come out of his home during noontime and call out for anyone who is hungry to please come and take the food. Only if no one comes in answer to his call can the chief of the household take his meals. There are so many rules and regulations just to train a man to become godly. They are not superstitious or superfluous. The human being should be trained to be godly. Because he is part and parcel of God, he is given the chance to be trained. This training is given because some day or other the person may be Kṛṣṇa conscious.

If by chance during this training he meets a teacher who is a saintly person and a pure devotee of the Lord, then by such a contact he becomes pure. Therefore, Lord Caitanya said that the fortunate person who has had some spiritual asset in his past dealings will seek the association of a pure devotee. The seed of Kṛṣṇa consciousness is received by the mercy of *guru,* the spiritual master, and by the mercy of Kṛṣṇa. When the spiritual master and Lord Kṛṣṇa will that a person must have Kṛṣṇa consciousness, then the seed very nicely fructifies. That spiritual asset makes one fortunate, and thus he becomes spiritually enlivened, and then he meets a bona fide spiritual master, and, by the grace of the spiritual master, he can receive the seed of Kṛṣṇa consciousness. That is his inner urge: "Where can I get this association? Where can I get this awareness?"

This process is recommended; it is the general process of spiritual advancement. Kṛṣṇa is within you, and as soon as Kṛṣṇa sees that you are very sincere, that you are seeking, He sends a bona fide spiritual master. This combination of Kṛṣṇa and the spiritual master is the cause of one's receiving the seed of Kṛṣṇa consciousness. The seed is there. If you have a very nice seed of a rose bush, what is your duty? If you have a seed of any nice plant, it is your duty not to lock it up in the safety vault of a bank. Your duty is to sow it in the ground. Where should you sow that seed? If you have information of Kṛṣṇa consciousness, you just sow it in your heart. Not in this earth, but in the earth within yourself. And after sowing a seed you have to pour a little water on it, so that water is hearing and chanting. Once the seed is sown in the heart, just pour on a little water, and it will grow.

This process should not be stopped by the thought that because one is initiated there is no need of hearing and chanting. It should go on continuously. If you stop pouring water on a plant, it will dry up; it will not produce any fruit. Similarly, even if you are highly elevated in Kṛṣṇa consciousness, you cannot stop this process of hearing and chanting because *māyā* is so strong, so powerful, that as soon as she sees, "Ah, here is an opportunity," at once you will dry up. By the process of pouring water, that plant of Kṛṣṇa consciousness grows. How does it grow? There is a limit to every plant you see; it grows and grows and grows, but there is a limit where it stops growing. But the plant of Kṛṣṇa consciousness grows in such a way that it does not rest in any part of this material universe because a Kṛṣṇa conscious person is not satisfied with planetary facilities in any part of this material universe. Even if you offer him Siddhaloka, where the inhabitants are so powerful and elevated that they can fly in the sky without airplanes, he will not be satisfied.

There is a planet, Siddhaloka, according to *Śrīmad-Bhāgavatam,* where the inhabitants do not need airplanes or spacecraft to fly from one planet to another. Above Siddhaloka there are many other planets. I saw that the latest modern opinion is that every star is a sun, and there are different planetary systems, solar systems; but according to Vedic literature there are innumerable universes which are separate identities. The limit of this universe is the outermost sky. The modern scientist says that each and every star is a sun. But Vedic literature does not say that. Vedic literature informs us that there is only one sun in each universe, but there are innumerable universes, and thus there are innumerable suns and moons. The highest planet of this universe is called Brahmaloka. And Lord Kṛṣṇa says, "Even if you approach the highest planet, you have to come back again." Sputniks and astronauts are going very high, and here on earth people are clapping; but after just a brief time they come down again. However one may clap, he cannot do more than that. Similarly, those who are materialistic can go high up to Brahmaloka where Brahmā is, but those who are Kṛṣṇa conscious will reject even that. They neglect even the impersonal *brahmajyoti*. They don't care for it.

The covering of this universe is far, far greater than this space which we are now in. The outside of the universe is ten times the space within, so one has to penetrate that covering, and then reach Virāja, the Causal Ocean. The Buddhist philosophical perfection is to reach that Virāja. When this material existence is completely finished, it is called *virāja*, according to Vedic language. But the Kṛṣṇa conscious person not only penetrates the covering of this universe, but after he reaches that Causal Ocean, which is the neutral position, he continues. The plant grows so nicely from Brahmaloka to Virāja to the spiritual sky, and even when that plant reaches the spiritual sky, it is not satisfied with any Vaikuṇṭha planet.

The highest planet in the spiritual sky is Kṛṣṇaloka. It is just like a lotus flower, where Kṛṣṇa is standing. And there, when the plant finds Kṛṣṇa's lotus feet, it rests. Just as a creeper grows and grows and grows and at last attaches itself to something and then expands, when the devotional plant gets to the lotus feet of Kṛṣṇa, it expands. As soon as this Kṛṣṇa consciousness creeper captures Kṛṣṇa's lotus feet, it takes shelter. "There. Now I have finished my journey. Let me expand here." To expand means to enjoy Kṛṣṇa's association. There the devotees are satisfied.

That creeper has to go on, and thus those who are already in Kṛṣṇa consciousness, if they have their natural growth, relish the fruit of that creeper even in this life.

If you continue this chanting and hearing process, you will grow and grow and actually reach Kṛṣṇa's lotus feet and there relish His association.

Glossary

Ahaṅkara—false ego, the junction point at which a person falsely identifies his self as the material body.

Ahaṁ Brahmāsmi—(lit.—"I am not this body; I am *Brahman*") Spiritual realization of the qualitative oneness of the infinitesimal individual with the infinite Supreme Lord Kṛṣṇa.

Bhakti-yoga—direct attachment to Kṛṣṇa.

Brahmacarya—student life of celibacy and study of *śāstras* under a spiritual master.

Brāhmaṇas—those trained in higher philosophical science, knowers of *Brahman* (spirit).

Kṣatriya—one trained and naturally qualified for ruling and for protecting the women, children, elderly persons and *brāhmaṇas.*

Mahāmantra—great chant for deliverance, the Hare Kṛṣṇa *mantra*.

Māyā—(lit.—"that which is not") Material atmosphere in which the conditioned soul tries to enjoy without Kṛṣṇa, or God.

Māyāvādīs—impersonalist philosophers who believe everything is illusion; they believe only in the impersonal aspect of God, but they do not recognize the source of the impersonal *Brahman,* the *Parambrahman,* or the Personality of Godhead.

Prasādam—food made spiritual by offering it to Kṛṣṇa.

Śāstra—scripture.

Śūdras—the laborer class who, by nature, serve others for their livelihood.

Vaikuṇṭha—where there is no anxiety; the spiritual world.

Vaiśyas—mercantile and agricultural class.

Yogeśvara—the master of *yoga*, the Supreme Lord Kṛṣṇa.

About Śrīla Prabhupāda

His Divine Grace A.C. Bhaktivedanta Swami Prabhupāda appeared in this world in 1896 in Calcutta, India. He first met his spiritual master, Śrīla Bhaktisiddhānta Sarasvatī Gosvāmi, in Calcutta in 1922. Bhaktisiddhānta Sarasvatī, a prominent religious scholar and the founder of sixty-four Gauḍīya Maṭhas (Vedic institutes) in India, liked this educated young man and convinced him to dedicate his life to teaching Vedic knowledge. Śrīla Prabhupāda became his student and, in 1933, his formally initiated disciple.

At their first meeting Śrīla Bhaktisiddhānta Sarasvatī requested Śrīla Prabhupāda to broadcast Vedic knowledge in English. In the years that followed, Śrīla Prabhupāda wrote a commentary on the *Bhagavad-gītā,* assisted the Gauḍīya Maṭha in its work, and, in 1944, started *Back to Godhead,* an English fortnightly magazine. Single-handedly, Śrīla Prabhupāda edited it, typed the manuscripts, checked the galley proofs, and even distributed the individual copies. The magazine is now being continued by his disciples in the West.

In 1950 Śrīla Prabhupāda retired from married life, adopting the *vānaprastha* (retired) order to devote more time to his studies and writing. He traveled to the holy city of Vṛndāvana, where he lived in humble circumstances in the historic temple of Rādhā-Dāmodara. There he engaged for several years in deep study and writing. He accepted the renounced order of life (*sannyāsa*) in 1959. At Rādhā-Dāmodara, Śrīla Prabhupāda began work on his life's masterpiece: a multivolume commentated translation of the eighteen-thousand-verse *Śrīmad-Bhāgavatam* (*Bhāgavata Purāṇa*). He also wrote *Easy Journey to Other Planets.*

After publishing three volumes of the *Bhāgavatam,* Śrīla Prabhupāda came to the United States, in September 1965, to fulfill the mission of his spiritual master. Subsequently, His Divine Grace wrote more than fifty volumes of authoritative commentated translations and summary studies of the philosophical and religious classics of India.

When he first arrived by freighter in New York City, Śrīla Prabhupāda was practically penniless. Only after almost a year of great difficulty did he establish the International Society for Krishna Consciousness, in July of 1966. Before he passed away on November 14, 1977, he had guided the Society and seen it grow to a worldwide confederation of more than one hundred *āśramas,* schools, temples, institutes, and farm communities.

In 1972 His Divine Grace introduced the Vedic system of primary and secondary education in the West by founding the *gurukula* school in Dallas, Texas. Since then his disciples have established similar schools throughout the United States and the rest of the world.

Śrīla Prabhupāda also inspired the construction of several large international cultural centers in India. The center at Śrīdhāma Māyāpur is the site for a planned spiritual city, an ambitious project for which construction will extend over many years to come. In Vṛndāvana are the magnificent Kṛṣṇa-Balarāma Temple and International Guesthouse, *gurukula* school, and Śrīla Prabhupāda Memorial and Museum. There is also a major cultural and educational center in Bombay. Major centers are planned in Delhi, Bangalore and a dozen other important locations on the Indian subcontinent.

Śrīla Prabhupāda's most significant contribution, however, is his books. Highly respected by scholars for their authority, depth, and clarity, they are used as textbooks in numerous college courses. His writings have been translated into over fifty languages. The Bhaktivedanta Book Trust, established in 1972 to publish the works of His Divine Grace, has thus become the world's largest publisher of books in the field of Indian religion and philosophy.

In just twelve years, despite his advanced age, Śrīla Prabhupāda circled the globe fourteen times on lecture tours that took him to six continents. Yet this vigorous schedule did not slow his prolific literary output. His writings constitute a veritable library of Vedic philosophy, religion, literature, and culture.